THE ART OF BALANCED LIVING

For Blake

THE ART OF BALANCED LIVING

The right diet and lifestyle
for your body type

DR SHAUN MATTHEWS

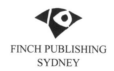

FINCH PUBLISHING
SYDNEY

The Art of Balanced Living: The right diet and lifestyle for your body type

First published in 2016 in Australia and New Zealand by Finch Publishing Pty Limited, ABN 49 057 285 248, Suite 2207, 4 Daydream Street, Warriewood, NSW, 2102, Australia.

17 16   8 7 6 5 4 3 2 1

There is a National Library of Australia Cataloguing-in-Publication entry available at the National Library.

Edited by Jenny Scepanovic
Editorial assistance by Megan English
Text designed and typeset by Meg Dunworth
Illustrations and diagrams by Meg Dunworth
Cover design by Jo Hunt

Printed by 1010 Printing

The paper used to produce this book is a natural, recyclable product made from wood grown in sustainable plantation forests. The manufacturing processes conform to the environmental regulations in the country of origin.

While every care has been taken with the research and compilation of the information in this book, it is in no way intended to replace a consultation with an appropriately qualified health care professional. Readers are encouraged to seek such help as they deem necessary. The author and publisher specifically disclaim any liability arising from the application of information in this book.

Finch titles can be viewed and purchased at **www.finch.com.au**

Contents

List of recipes

Introduction

We all know what it's like to feel balanced. Your muscles are relaxed, your mood is even and there is a sense of having energy to spare. Thoughts gently roll along and you are comfortably aware of both yourself and your surroundings. Though hard to put your finger on, there is a pervasive sense of wellbeing. Life is good.

So how can we create a way of being in the world where we feel balanced more of the time? A way of being that enables us to bounce back from the curve balls that life may throw at us, one that is both sustaining and sustainable?

This book addresses this question by drawing from the ancient wisdom traditions of India; traditions of wellbeing that were formulated many thousands of years ago that are as relevant today as they were at the time of their inception. Importantly they recognise that we are not all the same and, in simple terms, what works for one person may not work for another. Some of us do best with salads and raw foods while others require warm, cooked foods that are easy to digest. Some people come to life in cooler weather while others feel the cold intensely. Some of us love going for a run first thing in the morning while others prefer a long lie in or a slower start to the day.

What is presented here is an approach to understanding human beings that recognises constitutional difference and gives practical guidelines to help us stay more centred and relaxed from moment to moment. This book will introduce you to the body-typing system of Ayurveda, India's traditional system of healing, and how you can use its principles to better manage your health. It will show you how simple changes to your diet and lifestyle can bring you back to a state of balance and feeling better in yourself.

You will also learn how to care for your body, mind and spirit using practices and routines that create resilience and enhance wellbeing. The importance of finding that path through life that is supportive of both you and your community will also be explored, including how you can connect with that path.

Learning to live in tune with the flow of life is a central concern of Ayurveda and its sister sciences – yoga, meditation and Vedic astrology. In essence they address, both in theoretical and practical ways, that fundamental question for all of us: how do we live a life well lived? A life of meaning that satisfies our individual temperament, needs and aspirations, and which allows us to feel complete and whole at the time of its ending.

This question of how to live a life well lived was brought into sharp focus for me in my early twenties at a time of profound personal loss. Shortly after a family skiing holiday, my younger brother, who was travelling home a day early, was killed in a car accident. Numb with shock and disbelief, we stopped on our way home at the farm of some old friends. The next morning I woke early, instinctively knowing I needed to spend some time in the bush.

On a cold, bleak day with a light rain falling, I headed off in the half-light to a spot I knew in a large eucalypt forest. With the help of wallaby tracks and dried up creeks as landmarks, I eventually found the small clearing deep in the scrub country. It was here, after raging for some hours against the unreality of my brother's death, that the forest spoke to me. While lying on the wet ground beside a makeshift fire, I was opened to a panoramic view of life and death and blessed with the beginnings of a new understanding. An understanding that brought some solace in the midst of the utter desolation I felt.

I came to understand that the love I felt for my brother was not bound by time. Our lives in physical bodies might be subject to nature's cycle of birth, growth, decay and death, but the essential connection I felt with him is not. It was as if my intellect was pushed aside in that moment and a deeper knowing came through that spoke to my heart. The peace that I felt in that moment was to become a trusted guide in the journey ahead in my life, and led me to explore this thing called meditation; an intriguing word I had come across in novels by Herman Hesse.

I desperately wanted to stay true to what I had learnt that day in the forest and was concerned that it would be easy to get caught up in the sometimes petty and shallow concerns of daily living. Intuitively I felt that a daily practice of meditation would help me stay connected to the timeless dimension of life.

Several months later, while completing my final year of medicine, I was presented with the opportunity to learn how to meditate. With my best friend at the time, who also shared an interest in meditation, I undertook a course over several nights in transcendental meditation. Our teacher, a young woman in her thirties, radiated a sense of calm and inspired us through her words and presence. So began my initiation into the ancient wellbeing traditions of India, traditions that have since become an integral part of my daily life and enriched my practice of medicine.

My intention in writing this book is to help make these practices more available to Western audiences. It is one of the many paradoxes of our times that despite better education and health care, rates of obesity and diabetes are soaring. We enjoy unparalleled levels of personal freedom and yet more and more people are suffering from loneliness and depression. While modern science has given us mobile phones, the internet and cheap international travel, many feel disconnected from themselves and others and seem to have lost their way.

It is also true that we live in an age of extraordinary opportunity: the opportunity to escape rigid social conventions from the past and to start afresh, to create meaningful lives for ourselves where we can draw from the very best of cultural and spiritual traditions from around the world. In essence, to redefine what matters most to us in our lives and to construct ways of being that are in sync with those values. Whether it is what we choose to eat for breakfast, what type of work we engage in or how we manage our day-to-day stress, we are freer than ever to cultivate new ways of doing and being.

This book presents some of the basic tenets of ancient traditions of wellness to those who are eager to create a truly nourishing life for themselves. Traditions that value individual, community and planetary wellbeing and strive to live in harmony with Mother Nature.

Ayurveda focuses on how to establish a stable platform for physical, emotional and mental health through establishing a healthy diet and lifestyle. Astrology gives us guidance on how to live to our full potential, and yoga and meditation give us tools to manage our bodies and minds and to explore the spiritual dimension of life. As you might expect, there is considerable overlap between these traditions, as they are inextricably intertwined and complement each other.

Essentially, the traditions outlined in this book need to be lived in order for their value to be recognised and appreciated. All that is required is some degree of openness and a willingness to give them a go. It is in the doing of them that they begin to speak to you. Practise is an essential ingredient as it allows you to build up your own experience of what is being advocated. What begins as an external resource, over time becomes an internal resource that you can draw upon in your journey through life.

I also want to show that these principles of wellbeing can be integrated into a modern Western lifestyle with relative ease and that it is not necessary to live like a Zen monk in order to benefit from them. Importantly many of these traditions were designed for the householder, living in a family setting and engaged in secular life and, as such, are eminently suitable for people living a contemporary lifestyle.

I include in each chapter accounts from people who are already reaping the benefits of introducing some of these principles into their daily life. The individuals who generously share their experiences are patients, students and colleagues of mine, many of whom have experienced profound transformations in their physical and mental health and their enjoyment of life through a changed approach to living. An approach based around a view of life quite different from the one they were born into and which sees them taking on practices quite alien to mainstream Western culture.

The Appendices include easy-to-follow eating programs for the three body types of Vata, Pitta and Kapha; recipes that pacify the three doshas; and a selection of my favourite recipes that are balancing for all body types. And you can flick to the Glossary at the end if you come across any unfamiliar words.

I have chosen those principles that I feel are the most relevant to the art of balanced living. My selection is by no means exhaustive, and is tempered by the experiences I have had with my students and patients over the last 25 years. The chapters in this book are, by their nature, only an introduction, though it is my hope that they can serve as a useful bridge for those looking to deepen their enquiry into how to live an inspired and inspiring life. The Further reading and Resources sections at the end of the book are good starting points if you want to explore these ideas further.

I invite you to take this opportunity to test some of the principles presented in this book against your own lived experience and see whether they deserve to have a place in your life.

chapter 1

Identifying your body type

Vata, Pitta and Kapha are the three doshas, they give life to the body and destroy it, in their natural and disturbed states respectively.

Ashtanga Hridaya, Ayurvedic medical text

On a cool winter's morning at my local beach, a couple of swimmers emerge from the sea pool having completed their daily routine of 40 laps. Even though the outside temperature is 12 degrees Celsius and the water temperature only a few degrees above that, they are smiling broadly and glowing with vitality. Meanwhile, on the promenade above the pool, several walkers in tracksuits and woollen jumpers are watching the swimmers with a look somewhere between awe and bewilderment as if to say, 'How on earth do they do it? Are they mad?'

The fact that we are all different seems to marry with our common experience. Why is it that some of us can eat like a proverbial horse and lose weight, while others only have to sniff a lettuce leaf to put on weight? Why do some people struggle with constipation throughout their lives and others have two to three easy bowel motions a day? How is it that some people sleep soundly and deeply for eight hours a night, while others take a long time to get to sleep and wake at the slightest sound?

Our inherent differences are well recognised in the ancient traditions of India. Ayurveda, in particular, addresses this question directly and in an eminently practical way through an understanding of body type. It identifies three basic body types which, when properly understood, provide a wonderful key to creating a diet and lifestyle that is in keeping with your own unique nature. It also helps you to accept yourself as you are, not as you think you should be, when comparing yourself to others.

In this chapter, I introduce the basic principles of body type in Ayurveda and explain how you can use this knowledge to inform your approach to living life in harmony with your essential nature.

The seers of ancient India, known as rishis, are said to have asked the question, 'How can we know the universe?' They reasoned that ultimately we experience the world through our five senses. They posited a specific element for each of our five senses – the five elements being earth, water, fire, air and space. These five elements correspond directly to the five senses of smell, taste, sight, touch and hearing respectively.

This elemental way of viewing individuals is not as alien as it might seem. We all know people who are earthy – solid, dependable and grounded; people who are fiery – passionate, hotheaded and quick to anger; and people who are spacey – who seem to live with their heads in the clouds, immersed in a world of creativity and imagination. Ayurveda takes this basic idea one step further and looks at how your individual nature can be understood in terms of the interplay of these five elements.

The five elements are themselves the basis for three body-mind principles known as doshas. The word dosha does not have an easy English translation, but it is, in essence, an energetic phenomenon. We can understand the nature of each of the three doshas through its elemental composition:

- Vata dosha is derived from the elements air and space.
- Pitta dosha is derived from fire and water.
- Kapha dosha is derived from earth and water.

All living systems, including human beings, are seen as an expression of the interplay between these three doshas – Vata, Pitta and Kapha. Each dosha governs specific mental and physical processes in our bodies. Vata dosha is responsible for movement, Pitta dosha for transformation and Kapha dosha for cohesion.

How the doshas relate to our five senses

How we think, feel and act is a reflection of the relative amounts of the three doshas in our body type. In this way, differences in each person's nature can be understood and this knowledge used to create harmony and balance as we move through each day.

In Ayurveda, human beings are seen as part of nature, as much as plants and other animals are. So in order to live in harmony with nature, it helps if we can live in harmony with our own nature. By understanding your own individual nature more clearly, you are able to make conscious decisions about your diet and lifestyle in line with your natural tendencies.

IN AYURVEDA, HUMAN BEINGS ARE SEEN AS PART OF NATURE, AS MUCH AS PLANTS AND OTHER ANIMALS ARE.

Your body type determines your physical, emotional and mental tendencies. At the physical level, it will have a bearing on how you walk, your skin type, the kind of weather you feel most comfortable in and how your digestion functions. At the emotional level, it will have a bearing on how you react to people and situations, how you tend to resolve conflict and even how you deal with stress. At the mental level, it will have a bearing on how you approach tasks and process new information.

Ayurveda holds that your unique body type is determined at the moment of conception; the relative amounts of the three doshas in your body type are determined by the force of the doshas in your parents at the time of conception. Your body type does not change during your lifetime.

As with any system of typology, the Ayurvedic approach to viewing different constitutions can be used to enrich or diminish our view of ourselves and others. Certainly from an Ayurvedic perspective we are all seen as unique individuals, but it is also possible to identify distinct patterns of behaviour and innate tendencies in human beings. Used wisely, the Ayurvedic approach to body type is a powerful tool that can give us profound insights into human nature, allowing us to see how other people are different from us. It can also help us to better understand our own physical and psychological nature, and to accept ourselves as we are, not as we think we should be.

Why is it that no matter what I do, I can't shift that last 5 kilos of weight? Why am I so sensitive to raw food, often getting excessive wind and bloating? Why do I get angry so quickly when others seem so relaxed? Why can't I tolerate hot spices while others seem to thrive on them? Why is going to the toilet to pass a bowel motion so fraught with difficulty for me when others seem to go effortlessly? As we shall see, these are all questions that are well understood through the Ayurvedic science of body type. And Ayurveda gives us a comprehensive toolkit to address these issues.

At this point, if you don't have some understanding of your doshic make-up, I suggest that you complete the following self-assessment form. When doing the assessment, it is important to answer in terms of your whole life, not just the last few years.

Ayurvedic body type self-assessment

On the chart on the next page, circle which of the following three options for each body type characteristic most accurately describes you. You will end up with a score out of 20 for each of the three doshas – Vata, Pitta and Kapha. (Note: you may circle more than one option.)

Tally up the scores out of 20 for Vata, Pitta and Kapha dosha. As an example, a person with a predominant Vata body type might score Vata 15, Pitta 7 and Kapha 8. It also happens that the scores might be evenly spread between two doshas; for example, you might score Vata 12, Pitta 11 and Kapha 6. It is important to remember that everyone has all three doshas in their body–mind make-up and that no-one is a hundred per cent of any one dosha. Once you have completed the assessment, draw up a visual representation of your doshic make-up using a bar graph.

	Vata dosha	Pitta dosha	Kapha dosha
Frame	thin	medium	heavy
Hair	dry, kinky	soft, straight	thick, oily
Teeth	irregular	yellow	big, white, strong
Appetite	variable	strong, excessive	slow, steady
Skin	dry, rough	fair, sunburn easily	thick, oily
Sweat	scanty	profuse	moderate
Elimination	constipated easily	soft, loose habit	slow, heavy bowel
Physical activity	very active	moderate	lethargic
Sex drive	variable	strong	steady
Mind	restless, 'spacey' at times	analytical, methodical	stable
Speech	speak quickly, talkative	concise, intense	slow, cautious
Personality traits	sensitive, highly strung	strong, forceful	patient, quiet
Emotional temperament	fearful, anxious	irritable, fiery	calm, easy going
Lifestyle	like spontaneity	plan and organise well	enjoy habits
Climate preference	warm, humid	cold	warm, dry
Memory	forgetful	sharp	slow but prolonged
Endurance	low	medium	strong
Dreams	fearful, lots of movement	violent, energetic	watery, romantic
Sleep	light, difficulty falling asleep	sound	heavy, prolonged
Finances	spend quickly	moderate	good money saver

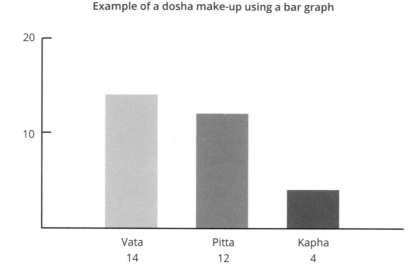

Example of a dosha make-up using a bar graph

The three body types in profile

Vata body type

If you have more Vata dosha in your constitutional make-up, you are likely to be thin and tend to lose weight when stressed. Your skin will be dry and you prefer warm weather and tropical climates. You may suffer from cold extremities, occasional constipation and digestive problems including burping, wind and a sensitive stomach. You tend to be more highly strung and run on nervous energy. Your mind is naturally very active and you like spontaneity. You approach life creatively but are prone to worry and anxiety. In your work you are attracted to creative fields including the arts, journalism and communication. Your challenge is not to take on too many things, which can overwhelm you and lead to depletion; the running-on-empty feeling.

An example of a Vata body type

Jacqui is a 32-year-old graphic designer who works for a women's magazine. Her weight fluctuates a lot depending on her stress levels and she tends to lose weight when feeling anxious. At work she is valued for her imaginative thinking and ability to get on with her fellow employees, especially when working in a team setting. She has a broad range of interests, loves theatre and dance and has a broad circle of friends. Jacqui has a tendency to take on too much, which can leave her feeling drained. If she is not careful with her diet or has too much raw food, she can suffer from excessive wind and bloating. It is important for her to get some form of exercise every day, which helps keep her feeling energetic and enthusiastic. She is a light sleeper and sometimes has difficulty getting off to sleep, especially if there is an important deadline at work.

Pitta body type

If you have more Pitta dosha in your constitutional make-up, you are likely to have a medium build and your weight tends to be constant, changing little over the years. Your skin will be fair and you can sunburn easily. You are sensitive to heat and prefer cold climates. You have a strong stomach but are prone to acidity and heartburn when stressed. You are insightful and have a strong capacity for discipline. You are dynamic, hardworking and focus well on tasks. You love being productive. You are ambitious by nature but are prone to frustration and workaholism. You are attracted to managerial and team leader positions and fields where your analytical capabilities are valued. The challenge for you is not to over-focus which can lead to overheating and burn-out.

An example of a Pitta body type
David is a 45-year-old project manager with an international IT corporation. At school he played competitive football and captained the school swimming team. He has a muscular body and prides himself on his personal fitness, which he maintains through jogging and regular gym workouts. His weight has changed little over the past 20 years. He enjoys skiing and surfing and finds tropical climates challenging. At work he is valued for his drive and leadership qualities and for his attention to detail. He loves taking on new challenges. He has a cast-iron digestion, though when stressed can suffer from heartburn and skin rashes. Over the years he has had a number of tendon and joint problems, especially when he pushes himself too hard when exercising. He is a sound sleeper.

Kapha body type

If you have more Kapha dosha in your constitutional make-up, you are likely to have a heavy build and can put on weight easily. Your skin is oily and your olive complexion tans easily. You prefer warm, dry weather and climates. You tend to be intolerant of high humidity. You have a sluggish digestion and are prone to mucus build-up in your chest and sinuses. You have good stamina and a calm, easy-going disposition. You perform tasks slowly and methodically. You are a steady worker and don't mind work that requires repetition. You have a caring and compassionate nature and are attracted to fields that allow you to nurture others such as nursing, hospitality and counselling. You are prone to stagnation, which can lead to melancholy and apathy. The challenge for you is to stay mentally stimulated and to maintain a physically active lifestyle; otherwise you can feel stuck in a rut.

An example of a Kapha body type

Paolo is a 50-year-old bank manager who has worked at the same bank since the age of 18. He is several kilos overweight and struggles to keep his weight down, despite trying various diets over the years. He is prone to comfort eating, which does not help. He tends to avoid exercise even though he knows it is good for him. He has an olive complexion and tans easily. At his bank branch, he is well liked by his employees for his calm and empathetic nature. His employers appreciate his methodical and thoughtful approach to his work. He is good in a crisis. He tends to avoid conflict, which has sometimes created problems for him, especially in his relationship with his wife. He enjoys relaxed time at home with his family and is an excellent cook. When stressed he is prone to colds and the occasional bout of bronchitis. He is a deep sleeper, but if he sleeps too much he can wake up feeling groggy.

The bi-doshic and monodoshic body types

Over the past 20 years in my medical practice, I have found that 40 per cent of the patients I see have one dosha dominant in their body type. This is known as a mono-doshic body type. In the other 60 per cent of patients, there is an fairly equal mix of two doshas present in the body type; what we call a bi-doshic body type. A body type where all three doshas are present in equal amounts is also described, though in my experience this is rare.

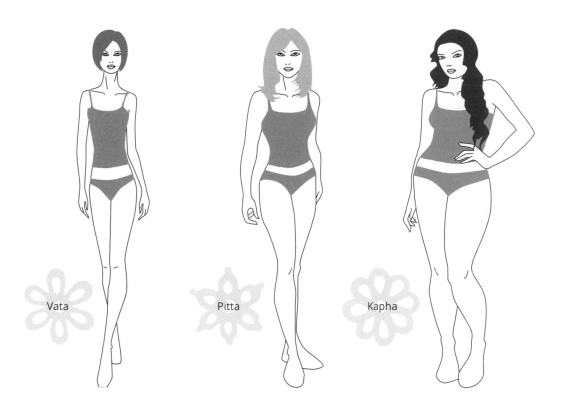

Vata Pitta Kapha

There are seven basic body types, as follows:

- Vata dominant body type
- Pitta dominant body type
- Kapha dominant body type
- Vata–Pitta body type
- Pitta–Kapha body type
- Vata–Kapha body type
- Vata–Pitta–Kapha body type.

A self-assessment form of this kind can be a useful starting point in understanding your Ayurvedic body type, though it does not replace a consultation with a well-trained and experienced Ayurvedic practitioner. If having completed this self-assessment, you are not seeing any recognisable pattern emerging, it is best to consult an Ayurvedic practitioner and request a body-type assessment. They will also be able to take your pulse, which gives valuable information in the determination of body type.

It is also true that your initial reaction to a situation can be helpful in working out your body type. This is well illustrated by the following teaching story used traditionally in India.

There are three people sitting in a room, one with a Vata body type, one with a Pitta body type and one with a Kapha body type. All of a sudden, a cobra slithers in through the door of the room. How will each person react? The person with the Vata dominant constitution, more fearful by nature, moves at lightning speed to the farthest corner of the room. The person with a Pitta dominant constitution, naturally courageous, will grab a chair and try and keep the snake at bay and kill it if necessary. The person with the Kapha dominant constitution, the most relaxed of the lot, sits still and lets someone else deal with the situation.

For readers wanting to further explore the question of their body type, I recommend Robert Svoboda's book *Prakruti: Your Ayurvedic Constitution*, which goes into considerable detail about the characteristics of the three mono-doshic body types as well as the bi-doshic body types.

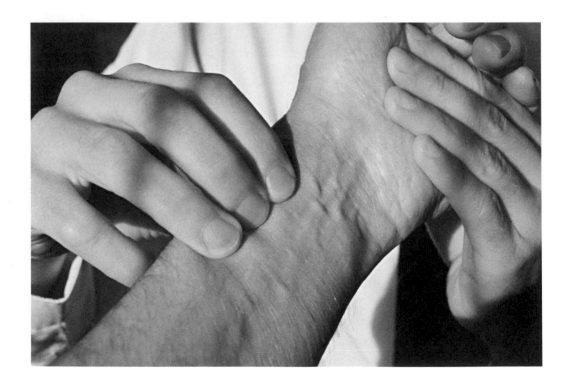

Chapter 2

Living in tune with your body type

One whose doshas are in balance, whose appetite is good, whose dhatus (tissues) are functioning normally, whose malas (waste products) are in balance. And whose physiology, mind and senses are always full of bliss, this is called a healthy person.

Sushruta Samhita, textbook of Ayurvedic surgery

Once you have a basic understanding of which dosha or doshas are dominant in your body type, you can begin to get a sense of what kind of food, drinks and activities are most likely to keep your doshas balanced. Balance is essentially a subjective experience, but we can say that when you feel balanced you generally feel relaxed and calm. Your digestion functions effortlessly, your mind is clear and your mood light. You are open to the present moment and whatever it may bring and there is a natural feeling of good will towards others.

The aim in Ayurveda is to keep you feeling like that more of the time as you travel through life, mindful that it is normal to experience ups and downs along the way. Feeling balanced engenders a quiet optimism and is, at heart, a very nurturing experience.

Doshas in and out of balance

When a dosha in our make-up is balanced it will express itself in a number of ways, including psychologically. When a person with a lot of Vata dosha in their nature is balanced, we experience them as enthusiastic, energetic, spontaneous, creative, flexible, quick thinking and open. The same person, when their Vata is aggravated, could feel agitated, anxious, insecure, spaced-out and prone to worry.

When a person with a lot of Pitta dosha in their nature is balanced, we experience them as warm, courageous, hardworking, insightful and engaging. When their Pitta is aggravated they are more likely to be angry, irritable, jealous, hypercritical, aggressive and obsessive. If they internalise this aggravated Pitta they can be resentful and perfectionist, becoming their own worst enemies.

By contrast, when a person with a lot of Kapha in their nature is balanced, we experience them as compassionate, calm, generous and easy going. The same person, if their Kapha dosha gets aggravated, could feel gloomy, depressed, apathetic and lethargic. They may be prone to greed, envy and possessiveness.

If we consider the different ways in which we respond to the experience of running late, we can learn more about how the doshas function when balanced and when out of balance. Someone whose Vata dosha is aggravated will worry and become anxious when running late for an appointment. Thoughts like, 'What if the other person doesn't wait for me and we miss each other?' or 'What will they think about my lateness? Will they be angry?' could be running through their mind. Someone whose Pitta dosha is aggravated will feel angry at the situation they have found themselves in and may try to blame someone or something else for their lateness. 'Why hasn't the traffic authority fixed this intersection yet?' or 'Why didn't I leave 15 minutes earlier? I knew the traffic would be bad.' Someone whose Kapha dosha is aggravated will feel flat or melancholic when running late for an appointment. 'I knew this would happen. I always seem to run late,' or 'I'm not good with time. This always happens to me,' are the thoughts they may be thinking.

When confronted with the experience of running late, the different body types react to the situation in ways consistent with their dominant dosha. By contrast, someone whose doshas are balanced is more likely to accept the fact that they are

> WHEN A DOSHA IN OUR MAKE-UP IS BALANCED IT WILL EXPRESS ITSELF IN A NUMBER OF WAYS ...

running late and respond in a calm and practical way. They will ring the other person, apologise for their lateness and tell them when they are likely to get there. Rather than punishing themselves or someone else for their predicament, they are more able to embrace the situation for what it is, without any undue fuss or drama.

Aggravated doshas: what they look like

❋ Vata – dry skin, constipation, joint or muscle pain, feeling cold internally, agitated, flighty, nervous, anxious, feeling insecure, running-on-empty feeling, talking quickly, excessive wind or bloating, diarrhoea.

❋ Pitta – red skin rash, heartburn, hyper-acidity, burning sensation, feeling hot internally, too intense, over-focused, impatient, angry, irritable, intolerant, aggressive, resentful, perfectionist, rage, jealousy, obsessive.

❋ Kapha – clammy skin, water retention, excessive mucus, weight gain from fat build up, apathetic, melancholic, flat mood, gloomy, greedy, possessive, stuck-in-a-rut feeling.

The principle of like increases like

Ayurveda utilises the principle of like increases like in its approach to keeping our doshas balanced. Through understanding the qualities or attributes of a substance or activity, we can see how it will affect our doshas. As Vata dosha is cold, light, dry, rough and mobile – reflecting its elemental composition – food that is cold, light, dry and rough will tend to increase Vata dosha. If we have a lot of Vata in our body type, eating this kind of food over a long period of time will tend to aggravate our Vata dosha.

In the case of Pitta dosha – which is hot, intense, slightly oily, sharp and penetrating – eating lots of hot, spicy, strong-tasting food over a long period of time will tend to aggravate our Pitta dosha.

Similarly, as Kapha dosha is cold, heavy, oily and soft, having lots of food with these qualities, such as dairy products and stodgy food will tend to aggravate our Kapha dosha.

The qualities of the three doshas

Vata	Pitta	Kapha
cool	hot	cold
light	intense	heavy
dry	slightly oily	stable
mobile	penetrating	soft
rough	sharp	oily

Using this principle, we can see that cold, windy weather, travel, irregular routines and too much fasting will increase Vata dosha. If we already have a lot of Vata in our nature, these things could potentially aggravate our Vata dosha, whereas hot, humid weather, too much work and not enough down time will potentially aggravate your Pitta dosha. If Kapha is dominant in your nature, then cold, damp weather, lack of exercise and overeating will potentially aggravate your Kapha dosha.

Generally speaking, the dosha or doshas that are most dominant in your nature are the ones that will cause you the most concern in your life. As they are present in greater amounts, it doesn't require as much to increase and then aggravate them. Below is a list of foods, drinks and activities that increase Vata, Pitta and Kapha doshas.

Vata
- Irregular eating and excessive fasting
- Loud noise and music
- Too much stimulation, especially TV, computers
- Violence and trauma of all kinds
- Eating light, cold and dry food
- Cold and iced drinks
- Late nights and lack of sleep
- Travel, especially high-speed travel
- Cold draughts
- Worry, anxiety

Pitta

- Eating hot, spicy and oily food
- Exposure to violence and aggression
- Excessive exposure to the hot sun
- Too much competition
- Too much conflict
- Anger, frustration
- Strong and bright lights
- Excessive alcohol and marijuana intake
- Intensity

Kapha

- Overeating
- Eating heavy, oily and stodgy food
- Too much sleep, especially during the day
- Comfort eating
- Sedentary lifestyle
- Lack of exercise
- Grief, sadness
- Too much routine in one's life
- Air-conditioning
- Lack of stimulation

Staying in balance

Our doshas are constantly in a state of flux depending on our diet and lifestyle, and are influenced by the weather, our state of mind and our emotions. While the basic amounts of the doshas are set at conception, it is also true that our doshas can go out of balance and become aggravated by certain factors.

Generally Ayurveda advocates moderation in all things. In this our bodies are our greatest allies, as they are constantly giving us information on how we are travelling. The challenge, given the busy lives that many people live in the 21st century, is to actually listen to what our bodies are saying.

Those foods, drinks and activities that make us feel good are to be encouraged and welcomed into our lives, whereas those things that make us feel poorly are to be avoided. Using these criteria, we can then create habits in our lives that really work for us, and which over time become second nature. As we do not always have control over the people, places, food and activities that we are engaging in, we can, at least, counterbalance those activities that have a negative effect on our wellbeing. In this way we have practical tools to neutralise the negative effects of certain influences on our lives, enabling us to retain our vitality and mental equilibrium.

Vata dosha responds well to warmth, stillness, nourishment and grounding; having a quiet day at home, catching up on your sleep, having regular meals and plenty of downtime. By downtime, I mean time where you are not 'doing' a lot; perhaps going for a gentle walk, or lying on your bed and connecting with yourself. This can be facilitated by gentle yoga stretches, calming breathing exercises, meditation that encourages relaxation and other self-care practices such as self-massage with oil. It tends to involve keeping your own company and not getting too stimulated by your environment. Warm, moist and easy-to-digest foods such as soups and casseroles in moderate amounts help us to feel more grounded.

... PEOPLE WHO HAVE DOMINANT PITTA DOSHA IN THEIR BODY TYPE CAN BECOME OVER-FOCUSED ...

Pitta dosha responds well to coolness and calmness and having fun; reducing the intensity of how you are living your life – not trying to pack so much into each day but having a more leisurely approach to life. A classical Ayurvedic text recommends taking walks under the moonlight with garlands of flowers around your neck with your partner. As people who have dominant Pitta dosha in their body type can become over-focused, especially with work, activities that are playful and encourage you to smell the roses are beneficial. It is also important for Pitta dosha types to drink plenty of fresh, non-chilled water and consume foods that are cooling in nature. Walks nearby to large bodies of water (rivers, lakes and the sea) and in nature are especially recommended.

Kapha dosha responds well to stimulation; this might be in the form of vigorous exercise, spicy food and new experiences through reading, travel and education. As people with more Kapha in their nature can easily become couch potatoes, a physically active lifestyle works well for them – activities such as bushwalking, jogging and sports that encourage them to extend themselves. Kaphas can also have a tendency to hold onto emotions and stew on them, so people and situations that encourage them to express their feelings and emotions are beneficial. Sleeping during the day is best avoided, as is eating stodgy food, both of which are a recipe for weight gain.

Living with a Vata-dominant body type

Ayurvedic principles have been practically useful to Emilee, a 30-year-old beauty therapist, who has completed a 12-week introductory course in Ayurveda for self-healing.

Through my exploration of Ayurveda and Vedic traditions, I have found that I have strong Vata traits, including the Vata tendency to disengage with the body, spending too much time in the head, which can often lead to anxiety and unnecessary worry. Recognising this in myself, I was keen to find ways to release negative energy and emotion, and clear my mind so I can remain centred and fulfilled. Grounding activities such as meditation and yoga have been extremely helpful for me in calming my mind and maintaining engagement with my body as well as teaching me to remain present in life and not get carried away with scattered thoughts.

Learning about the connection between my mind and body also taught me the concept of nourishing my dosha through nutrition in order to maintain balance. Another change I have incorporated is eating smaller meals more regularly instead of allowing my Vata tendency of becoming so engrossed in tasks I forget to eat. This has improved my balance greatly.

I have also found that increasing oil in my diet, massaging slightly warmed oil into my skin and burning aromatherapy oils such as lavender and rose have also been useful in supporting my dosha and maintaining balance and calming the mind, particularly when I am feeling cold or out of sorts.

Ayurveda also reignited my desire to remain connected to my spiritual side through Vedic principals. The concept of living in accordance with your dharma (your path), and how being aligned with your dharma can nourish your heart and, in turn, the hearts of those around you, has also been of great interest to me.

Implementing these small changes into my everyday life has made a huge impact on my personal experience in the world.

Balancing the three doshas – a practical guide

Balancing Vata dosha

- Sitting still, meditating, relaxing and sleep
- Eating warm, heavier, moist foods that are grounding in nature
- Eating foods cooked with warming spices such as ginger and cinnamon
- Self-massage with sesame oil or seeing your favourite masseur or masseuse
- Avoiding cold draughts or winds
- Wet saunas
- Staying at home rather than being out and about
- Wearing clothes that are pink, yellow, orange and white in colour
- Slow and calming yoga practice

Balancing Pitta dosha

- Not being so intense about whatever it is that you are doing
- Maintain plenty of leisurely pastimes
- Having fun, playing with children, walking the dog
- Food that is cooling in nature
- Reduce or avoiding hot, spicy foods and very salty foods
- Cooling and bitter herbs such as coriander, fennel and radicchio
- Avoid alcohol, recreational drugs and coffee
- Drinking plenty of fresh, non-chilled water
- Swimming and walks by the sea
- Wear cooling colours such as green, blue, grey, purple and white
- Cooling yoga practice

Balancing Kapha dosha

- ◉ Food that is light, dry and less oily in nature
- ◉ Food cooked with warming spices such as garlic, ginger, mustard, black pepper and chilli
- ◉ Occasional fasting or taking two meals a day
- ◉ Avoid too much sleeping especially after meals and during the day
- ◉ Avoid eating for emotional comfort
- ◉ Dry saunas
- ◉ Wear warm and stimulating colours, such as pink, yellow, orange and violet
- ◉ Avoid air conditioning, if at all possible
- ◉ Vigorous and stimulating yoga practice

 ## Living with a Pitta-dominant body type

Bryan, a 65-year old man who works as a business development director, shares how having an understanding of his body type has been useful to him.

My constitution is a mixture of Pitta and Kapha dominated by Pitta, however, I'm prone to Vata aggravation. My constitution provided an explanation for the cause of my IBS as well as my tendency to become overweight and depressed.

The biggest benefit I (continue to) get from Ayurveda is a deeper knowledge of self. My Pitta constitution explained my love for pilchards in hot chilli sauce when I was in my teens. It explained my excessively oily scalp, my thin, fair hair and my baldness that started at the age of seventeen. It also provides an explanation for how I can become obsessed with topics and how I get super critical of myself and others when my constitution is out of balance.

It's a great relief to know that my behaviour is not totally due to my personality but is influenced by my prevailing constitution and that this can be changed by altering my diet and lifestyle, with assistance from Ayurvedic herbs when needed.

The Pitta constitution also has benefits. I started swimming at the end of summer and because I intended to keep swimming throughout winter, I bought a wet suit. But I found that even though the temperature of the water fell to around 15 degrees Celsius I didn't need my wetsuit! I seem to handle lower temperatures really well.

Living with a Kapha-dominant body type

Ali, a 41-year-old wife, energetic helper and mother with two children shares her experience of having a Kapha dominant body type.

As a Kapha, I have excess mucus in the form of post-nasal drip or the feeling of mucus running down the back of my throat and feeling like I need to constantly clear my throat. When I have dairy, the symptoms are aggravated. Using a neti pot cleanse with warm, salty water in the shower is useful for this. Also useful are some aromatherapy oils such as peppermint in a diffuser or rubbed on my throat area.

I can identify with the sluggishness and stagnation of an out-of-balance Kapha – particularly when it comes to exercise. For me, a strong and disciplined routine is essential. I have the strength and endurance qualities of a Kapha – it is just getting past that warming-up phase. I feel that I innately hold back energy and keep some ready for endurance.

Having a slow digestive fire is another Kapha trait that I have observed – as well as a slow metabolism and holding onto excess weight and fluid. I try to add spices and heat to most of my meals – like chilli flakes, chilli sauce or cayenne pepper as a condiment – which has helped to heat up my digestion. Ginger has also been very useful in cooking and drinking hot water as a tea. And eating a smaller meal or spicy soup at night has been useful.

Being a Kapha I really feel the cold, but with the right preparation winter has been far more bearable.

When I am out of balance physically I also notice the emotional impacts – being lethargic, emotionally flat, a bit on the pessimistic side and stagnated. Sometimes it is hard to get myself out of this state – once again it is all about the disciplined routine – exercise, eating foods that agree with me, as well as practising yoga and meditation. Self-massage with sesame oil has been useful in my daily regime to get the circulation going as well as to warm up.

I have also realised that is not helpful for me to sleep in. As a Kapha it is optimal for me to get up at sunrise and I have more energy if I do that. Mid-afternoon is also another time when I feel like a nap. That is when I need to get active by cleaning or doing something physical to get my body moving.

The three body types in relationships

The first thing to say on this subject is that when you are in a state of balance, you are best equipped to meet the challenge of maintaining a happy and satisfying relationship. Whether it is with your partner, your parent, your child, a friend or a work colleague, being in balance is likely to make you less reactive and more understanding of the inevitable conflict that arises in the context of relationships.

Understanding how other people are innately different to you and how their behaviour may well be an expression of their body type can be extremely useful in negotiating the challenges of relationships. For example, individuals with more Pitta in their nature tend to be interested in detail. Once you understand that aspect of their nature, you will be less likely to be irritated by what you might see as their pernickety tendencies and more able to see that this is simply an expression of their body type. It becomes easier not to take things personally and embrace how people see and do things differently to you.

... BEING IN BALANCE IS LIKELY TO MAKE YOU LESS REACTIVE AND MORE UNDERSTANDING ...

People with more Kapha in their nature can sometimes be quite blunt in how they express themselves. This can potentially be quite hurtful to a naturally sensitive, Vata-dominant person. However, once they know that this is just how a Kapha-dominant person communicates, rather than viewing their comment as insensitive, they can see it for what it is and no offence need be taken.

People with more Vata in their nature often struggle with routine, resulting in an erratic and sometimes chaotic approach to life. As like increases like, when two Vata individuals get together, these tendencies can become stronger. By contrast, a Vata-dominant individual can often benefit from association with a Pitta-dominant person who likes to have more control in their life and has a natural capacity for discipline. That same Vata-dominant individual could also find the slow and steady approach of a Kapha dominant person helps keep them grounded and calmer.

As Vata-dominant individuals are more prone to worry and anxiety, they will often find the courage and confidence of a Pitta-dominant person very reassuring. Similarly people with more Vata dosha in their nature will benefit from the calm and naturally compassionate qualities of a balanced Kapha-dominant person.

Vata dominant individuals are blessed with a quick and creative mind and the ability to see the big picture. If paired with the focused and detail-oriented mind of a Pitta-dominant person when working on a project together, it can potentially be very frustrating for both of them. This is where recognising the innate differences of the three body types can help in accepting the other person's approach rather than generating tension in the relationship.

Differences between the body types can play out on many levels. One elderly couple I knew found it difficult to go for walks together in the park. She had more Vata in her nature and liked to walk quickly; he had more Kapha in his nature and liked to slowly amble along. Eventually, a compromise was found, whereby she would walk ahead of him and then come back and walk with him for a while, so that they could enjoy some time walking together. Here the naturally adaptable Vata individual found a way to manage their differences.

> DIFFERENCES BETWEEN THE BODY TYPES CAN PLAY OUT ON MANY LEVELS.

People with more Pitta in their nature have a natural intensity in how they approach life. They can become over-focused on the task at hand and have difficulty separating themselves from their current project. As such, they are more prone to becoming workaholics and forgetting to take breaks and holidays. In this instance, it is helpful for these Pitta dominant people to associate with people with more Vata dosha in their nature who can get overwhelmed by too much intensity and enjoy diversions and creative outlets. People with more Kapha who like to conserve their energy and have a nurturing disposition can moderate the drive of the Pitta-dominant person, helping them from burning themselves out.

As individuals with more Pitta in their nature can be willful and even arrogant at times, the influence of the naturally sensitive Vata person may help the Pitta-dominant person be more mindful of the effect of their actions on other people. The earthy pragmatism of a Kapha-dominant person may also serve to keep a naturally ambitious Pitta-dominant person more grounded and realistic about their plans.

People with more Kapha in their nature have great physical and mental stamina and patience. They are well able to last the distance with this combination of traits, long after Pitta-dominant types have given up in frustration and become burnt out, and Vata-dominant body types have simply lost interest and moved on to the next project that has captured their attention. As Kapha-dominant individuals tend to have stable minds, they can be relied upon in a crisis and are unlikely to do anything ill considered. This quality will appeal to Vata dominant individuals who can be prone to panic and flightiness, though they may find the Kapha dominant person's approach to situations somewhat boring and staid.

Kapha-dominant individuals can sometimes have difficulty in adapting to new situations. They may be perceived as stubborn and can have great difficulty changing their position on an issue. They need time to quietly think things through and will not be swayed by forceful coercion. Naturally this can frustrate Pitta-dominant individuals wanting to get things happening and Vata-dominant people who have already seen the big picture and are several steps ahead of them mentally.

People with more Kapha dosha in their body type are generous by nature, a trait not lost on Vata-dominant individuals, who are inclined to run on empty. When a Kapha cooks, they will cater for an entire football team and they are often much valued for their nurturing qualities. With their natural physical and mental resilience they are well able to carry an extra load, whether it is shopping bags at the supermarket or extra work in the office. Their capacity for empathy and compassion is much valued by people with Vata-dominant body types, who will feel safe and secure in their presence. By the same token, individuals whose predominant dosha is Pitta will be less inclined to be self-critical and hard on themselves when in the company of a person with plenty of Kapha dosha in their nature.

 Managing a bi-doshic body type

A colleague of mine in his sixties, who practises as a psychotherapist, shares his experience of having a bi-doshic body type.

I relate to having a Vata–Pitta body type, but I tend to suffer more from Vata disturbances than Pitta disturbances. I have travelled a lot in my life, live in the city and do a lot of mental work, all of which have increased my Vata dosha. Though when I was younger I suffered a lot of Pitta disturbances – fever, boils and diarrhoea.

I have a very spontaneous, creative mind. I think a lot, about a lot of different things but my Pitta gives me a lot of focus. I'm on the move a lot of the time and need to be physically active, which is the Vata aspect of my nature; from a Pitta perspective I enjoy exercises that have a martial arts aspect to them and that involve using my muscles.

I enjoy warmth, but I don't like when it is too hot. I do feel the cold because of the Vata in my body type. I have a very strong appetite, which is a Pitta trait and if I don't eat I become irritable. It's like a furnace. I don't put on weight at all. My digestion is strong enough to manage most foods.

My number one challenge with having a Vata–Pitta body type is staying still. The best thing for me is to take time out. My Pitta dosha drives me to consume, to be active and fuels my ambition. I have a disciplined lifestyle – my primary mode is having routine.

I slow down using yoga asanas and breathing practices and a lot of meditation. I find doing yoga nidra, a lying-down meditation practice, very important. I do that on a daily basis. Every morning I do asana or qigong and during the day I do breath-work. If I have a heavy day seeing a lot of clients, I will do yoga nidra between my afternoon and morning sessions. I find it very powerful. Between clients I will stretch or go for a gentle walk to help my circulation.

I find food very useful in balancing my body. I use a lot of grounding, warming and nourishing foods. I avoid cold foods, especially in winter. In winter I have a lot of oatmeal porridge and have recently been trying cooked quinoa flakes. I find eating regularly is very important for my wellbeing.

At night I do a lot of stretching and gentle meditation to calm the nervous system before bed.

The biggest challenge for me is not having a lot of stamina. I really value the spontaneity that comes with having more Vata dosha in my constitution, but I need to constantly manage it. I like the lightness and flexibility that comes with my body type, it's easy to be active and move around but there is also the challenge not to overdo it. As I get healthier I don't notice my doshas; they don't manifest so much.

I think the thing I value most about the Vata in my nature is the creativity and the Pitta is the ability to focus.

The three doshas in the kitchen

Your dominant dosha expresses itself in everything you do. How you walk, how you talk, the quality of your eye contact and even how you drive your car. It also determines your approach to preparing a meal and cooking. In this sense, watching individuals with different body types cook can be illuminating.

With Vata body types, it all happens quickly. Cooking tends to be a spontaneous affair and they enjoy experimenting with creative food combinations. Planning tends to be minimal, measuring of ingredients non-existent, and the whole process can have a somewhat chaotic edge, marked by a flurry of arm movements and racing around. It is easy for them to get distracted, which can adversely affect the final outcome and occasionally result in a burnt offering at mealtimes!

Pitta body types bring their powers of organisation to the process of meal preparation and tend to cook with great economy. As such, they will often prefer to clean up as they go. Their meals may lack the creativity and flair of a Vata type, but there will be less washing up at the end of the meal!

The Kapha types cook in a slow and steady manner, which can be very frustrating for Pitta types who need food NOW! If you have been invited to the home of a Kapha type you can be sure the meal will have been well researched and patiently planned, even if the execution meanders along. That said, Kapha types tend to be great lovers of food and drink and the meal will most likely be worth the wait.

Acknowledging differences in preference

Potential areas of mismatch among body types include how you start the day. Vata types often have a lot of energy early in the morning and enjoy jogging and being physically active at this time, whereas Kapha dominant types like to sleep in and then have a leisurely breakfast, preferably in bed!

Eating out can also present problems as Vata-dominant types like to experiment with new restaurants and are open to trying different cuisines. By contrast, Kapha-dominant types are more inclined to go to tried and tested restaurants that they know and trust. Pitta dominant types, when out of balance, seek out strong-tasting and spicy food that appeals to their need for intensity, although when they are more balanced they will naturally avoid too much chilli, which causes them to overheat.

Choosing a holiday destination can also present difficulties. Vata- and Kapha-dominant types love warmth, as they are essentially cold constitutions. Vata-dominant types revel in tropical environments, whereas Kapha dominant types may find the humidity uncomfortable and will prefer arid places. Pitta-dominant types do not tolerate warm and moist weather well and enjoy skiing, mountain walks and time near the ocean, which helps them stay cool and calm.

Travelling in a car over long distances can be challenging when there are different body types involved and finding the right setting on the air-conditioning unit can become a vexed issue. Pitta-dominant types will like the air-conditioning to be on full blast in summer, but this will be too cold for Kapha dominant and especially Vata dominant types. Too much heating in winter will bring out the explosive qualities of a person whose dominant dosha is Pitta, as they can't bear overheating.

When it comes to exercise, Kapha dominant types like to conserve their energy and can be prone to avoidance of physical activity, whereas Vata dominant types, assuming they have not allowed themselves to get run down, enjoy expending energy and can even be prone to exercise addiction. Pitta dominant types are generally good at managing their energy expenditure, but if they get too competitive they can burn themselves out and run into problems with fatigue in the long term.

TRAVELLING IN A CAR OVER LONG DISTANCES CAN BE CHALLENGING WHEN THERE ARE DIFFERENT BODY TYPES INVOLVED ...

The three doshas in bed

Sharing a bed with someone whose body type is different from your own can be a challenging affair. Consider the following situation: on a warm summer's night a couple have just retired to bed. Chloe, a Vata-dominant type who feels the cold easily, is snuggled up very happily under a lightweight doona. Meanwhile Frank, her Pitta-dominant partner, is already overheating. He has thrown off the doona and sheets and is stomping around the bedroom trying to set up a fan at the end of the bed. Sound familiar?

This is just another way that the dance of the doshas expresses itself. In general terms Vata types crave warmth. They will be sensitive to any cold drafts in the bedroom and will often need to wear woollen socks to help them to sleep. They do well with earplugs to reduce the impact of noise coming from the street or their partner, and benefit from wearing an eye mask to ward off the stimulating effect of the morning light. Sadly Vata types are often labelled neurotic by other body types, who do not understand their sensitive disposition.

For people with a dominant Pitta body type, it's all about finding the right temperature in bed. This can be a tricky affair especially if the ambient temperature changes through the night. A layered approach to bedding works best for them, allowing them to fine-tune the amount of warmth or coolness required in order for them to sleep soundly.

Kapha body types have a little more fat tissue in their make-up, so they tend to be less sensitive to temperature changes once they are in bed. They tend to be able to sleep for long periods of time, but can oversleep, which causes them to feel lethargic and groggy in the morning. They dislike humidity and benefit from electric fans, open windows and bedrooms with plenty of airflow.

On the sexual front, Vata-dominant types are quick to arouse but are prone to becoming depleted from too much sex. They need adequate time to rest and rejuvenate after sex. By contrast Kapha-dominant types, though slow to arouse, have a lot of sexual stamina and are said to be able to go all night! Pitta-dominant types tend to have a strong libido and are well able to get into action, however, they become angry if their desire is thwarted!

The three body types in children

As a parent, having an understanding of your child's body type can be very useful to better manage their physical and psychological wellbeing. I find there is often a strong correlation between what Ayurveda would recommend for an individual child and what your intuition as a parent is saying. It is also true that sometimes children will know intuitively what suits them best, if only the parent will listen to them!

I recently had a mother bring in her eight-year-old daughter for an Ayurvedic body type assessment and to get some advice about the most appropriate diet for her daughter. As it turned out, most of my recommendations, which involved having smaller, more frequent meals and more cooked food to suit her predominantly Vata body type, were very much in line with what her daughter had been requesting for some years.

In general terms, children with a predominant Vata body type are sensitive by nature and need to be treated gently. They are blessed with a strong imagination and are original thinkers, but can react to new situations in a fearful manner. They need daily, moderate exercise to help them stay connected to their bodies, are light sleepers and can sometimes have difficulty getting to sleep. Children with more Vata dosha in their nature respond well to a regular bedtime routine, and a foot massage before sleep can work wonders with them.

As Vata dosha is cold in nature, these children feel the cold and it is important that they are not under-dressed in cold weather, which will cause them to become scattered in their thinking and somewhat agitated. They tend to be fussy eaters, which can create challenges for their parents at mealtimes. Generally, they do well with smaller, more frequent meals and food which is warm and easy to digest.

Children with a predominant Pitta body type are strong-willed by nature and need to be treated firmly, as they like to dominate. They are natural leaders and enjoy being challenged. They are competitive in most situations, particularly on the sports field, though too much competition can aggravate their Pitta dosha. They become frustrated easily and care needs to be taken lest they take on something that is beyond their capability.

As Pitta is hot in nature, these children can be intolerant of hot weather and a cool, moist towel over their heads especially at bedtime is very soothing in summer. They have strong appetites and need to be fed promptly when they are hungry to avoid angry outbursts and tantrums. They do well with raw food and should be encouraged not to overeat.

THE BODY TYPE OF A CHILD EXPRESSES ITSELF FROM THE MOMENT THEY ARE CONCEIVED, ...

Children with a predominant Kapha body type are placid by nature and respond well to physical and mental stimulation. They are empathetic by nature, but can be slow to express their emotions. It is important to gently encourage them to express their feelings and for them to feel heard. They like to conserve their energy and can be prone to becoming lounge lizards, watching TV and playing computer games. Although they will resist it, they do well with plenty of exercise, which stops them becoming apathetic and lethargic.

Children with more Kapha in their nature tend to use food as comfort, which can lead to weight gain, especially if the food is high in fat and salt. Kapha dosha is heavy in nature, so eating light food such as steamed vegetables, rice crackers and leafy greens is recommended. They are often attracted to cheese and other dairy products, which will aggravate their Kapha dosha if taken in excess.

The body type of a child expresses itself from the moment they are conceived, and is evident from birth. Most parents, with some Ayurvedic knowledge, will be able to pick the dominant dosha in the body type of their child by the time they are six months old. I well remember attending a birthday party of a one-year-old where there were three one-year-old children present. It soon became clear that all three dosha types were represented. The little girl with more Vata in her nature was constantly moving around the room crawling over couches and pillows; the little boy with more Kapha in his nature sat in the middle of the room, never moving, with a lovely big smile on his face; while the boy with more Pitta in his nature was somewhere in the middle in terms of his energy levels, busy trying to catch up with the little girl and the first to get to the party food on offer!

The dance of the doshas

I encourage you to take your time in determining the dominant dosha or doshas in your body type. It takes a while to integrate these principles into your understanding of yourself. It is useful to imagine that you have a Vata-dominant constitution for one week and to view the world in that light. The following week imagine that you have a Pitta-dominant constitution, and then for another week, imagine that you have a Kapha-dominant constitution. With this experience under your belt you will then be better placed to see how the different doshas are operating in your life.

Health tip

A warm foot bath and gentle massage is a great way to help children get to sleep.

As you start to see how the energies of the three doshas play out in the different domains of everyday life, you will get a sense of whether the doshas are balanced or out of balance. With this information you can begin to manage your doshas by making changes to your diet and lifestyle and adopting self-care practices. By way of example, my partner and I went for a long walk on a cold and windy winter's day. Afterwards she felt unsettled and cold internally. Aware of the Vata aggravating nature of the weather, I suggested she take a long hot shower and give herself a warm oil massage, which she did. I also made her a cup of herbal tea that helped pacify the increase in her Vata dosha. She soon felt better both physically and mentally and was back to her normal self.

Looking at the world, including your own body, through the lens of the three doshas does require a little practice, but in my experience the dance of the doshas soon reveals itself. You begin to see how different foods, activities, and weather conditions make you feel – physically, emotionally and mentally. You can then frame your experience in terms of the three doshas. Am I feeling balanced or out of balance in some way? If I am feeling out of balance, which of the doshas seems to be involved – Vata, Pitta or Kapha?

With this knowledge, you can then set about putting yourself back on a path to balance, using those foods, drinks and lifestyle measures that will pacify the aggravated dosha. Over time, as you get to know yourself better and become more familiar with your patterns of imbalance, you are better placed to nip things in the bud before they get out of hand. In this way, you have a practical key to preventive health care and wellbeing.

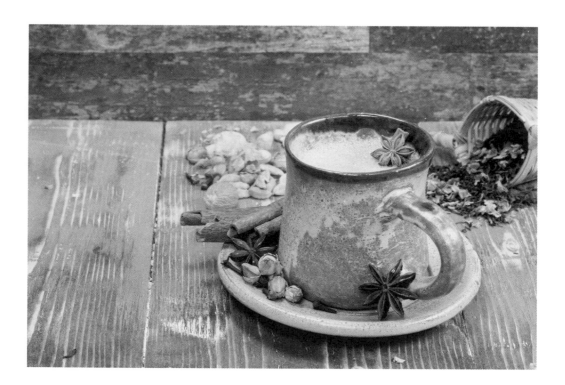

chapter 3

Maintaining a strong immune system

Even the wholesome food also taken in proper quantity, does not get digested due to anxiety, grief, fear, anger, uncomfortable bed and vigil.

Charaka Samhita, textbook of Ayurvedic medicine

It has long struck me how people have very particular preferences when it comes to breakfast. Our toast must be the right shade of brown, our tea must have the right amount of milk and our porridge must be the right consistency for us to enjoy it. My partner and I are no exception, and it is clear to me that our food choices for the first meal of the day strongly reflect our different body types.

My partner has a lot of Kapha dosha in her constitution, so the theme for her breakfast is stimulation. She will always begin with a strong espresso coffee, reflecting her continental background, to kick-start her day. This is very balancing to the Kapha tendency to stagnation. This will be followed by toast with no butter and thinly spread jam; the warmth and lightness of the toast is perfect for the cold and heavy nature of her constitution. As she has a Kapha body type, she knows how easily she can put on weight and so avoids too much dairy and sugar. If she does have cereal, it will be with skim milk and she will sprinkle a mixture of puffed amaranth, rolled oats and linseed over it to help keep her digestion balanced.

By contrast, I like a gentler start to the day where the theme is more about sustaining nourishment to get me through to lunch. I like nothing better than to begin with warm stewed fruit, especially apples or pears, on top of toasted muesli. The warmth and moistness of the fruit appeals to the Vata in my nature and the fibre in the muesli helps keep me regular. This is followed by toast with dollops of butter and thickly spread marmalade, which gives me energy and is filling. I have an active lifestyle and can lose weight if I don't eat regularly, so the fat and sugar is helpful. A cup of medium strength tea with full cream milk is a perfect nurturing end to breakfast for me.

Ayurveda recognises that we are not all the same and that different body types have different needs in order to stay balanced. This is certainly the case when it comes to the dietary requirements of the different body types, a subject I cover in some detail in Chapter 5. For now, I want to look at how the ancients viewed digestion and why it was seen as the key to good health.

Agni – your digestive fire

In the traditional medical systems of Europe, China and India, good digestion and strong immune system functioning go hand in hand, so great attention is given to the quality of food, how foods are combined, and how they are prepared and eaten. The sharing of food is seen as a sacred ritual that nourishes us on many levels, not just the physical.

By contrast, in our predominantly materialistic culture in the West, food and drink are viewed more as petrol that needs to be put into our tanks in order for us to have the energy to do the things we want to do. In our modern life is it is common for us to eat on the run, at the bus stop, driving to work and frequently standing up. TV dinners and practices such as eating and reading simultaneously are the norm and rarely questioned.

I would like to introduce you to another way of approaching digestion; a way that has far-ranging implications in preventing disease and in the promotion of mental and physical wellbeing. Through a better understanding of the process of digestion and through a sensitive listening to your body, you can start to manage your health more intelligently and responsibly.

In ancient India and continuing up to the present day, the transformative nature of fire has been worshipped and given a central role in the process of sustaining life. It is known as agni, which simply means fire in Sanskrit, though it exists in many forms. In terms of the human being, agni refers to our digestive capacity. To what extent are we able to draw nourishment from the food we eat? Does our diet make us feel energetic and nurtured or does it make us feel heavy and lethargic?

Agni also refers to our capacity to digest our life. If aspects of our life have been become indigestible, this will be mirrored in our physical digestion. If we are persisting in a toxic relationship that we know is no good for us or haven't fully grieved an intimate relationship that has broken up, then this will affect our agni. Chronic workplace dissatisfaction or long-term anxiety over money will also have an effect on our agni. In this way, the concept of agni recognises the inherent link between the quality of our thoughts and emotions and our physical body. All three are seen as part of an energetic whole: they are inextricably connected and influence each other.

How your agni cooks your food

Ayurveda makes use of a number of simple, naturalistic metaphors to explain complex physiological processes, that, in my experience, Western medicine is still struggling to understand. In the case of the agni, the digestive tract is seen as a pot in which our food and drink is mixed and cooked. If we have a balanced digestive fire, the contents of the pot are well cooked and transformed into a nourishing nutrient broth that is easily assimilated into the body. This broth, loaded with the right amounts of carbohydrates, fats, proteins, vitamins and minerals, is akin to the plasma in our blood. Plasma is the fluid portion of blood left over when red blood cells, white blood cells and platelets are removed from the blood.

In Ayurveda, the agni and immune system functioning are closely related. If the digestive fire has become weak, then the contents of the pot are not properly digested, this material is hard to assimilate and is said to block the channels of the body – that is, the blood vessels and lymphatic capillaries. If the fire has become

Managing the Agni

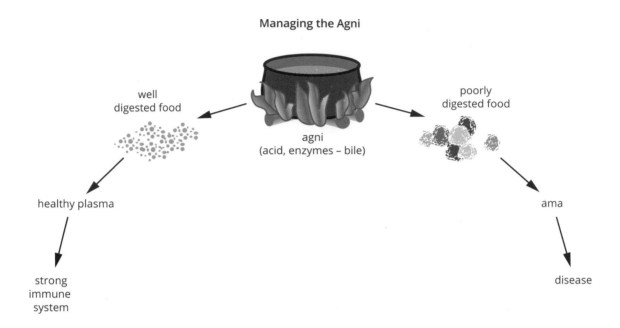

well
digested food

agni
(acid, enzymes – bile)

poorly
digested food

healthy plasma

ama

strong
immune
system

disease

very strong, then the contents of the pot can get burnt, which can also cause problems when that material enters into the bloodstream.

Improperly cooked, undigested food material is known as 'ama' in Ayurveda. It is held to be the root of all disease, as described in Sanskrit texts written two and a half thousand years ago. Ama tends to accumulate in tissues and organs, reducing the level of nourishment to that organ. Ayurveda posits that each of us has a weak link in our bodies, and that ama will tend to affect those tissues or organs the most, thereby impairing immune system functioning. As we know from common experience, when under prolonged stress some people will come down with bronchitis, others may get a migraine and still others may get a stomach ulcer.

Agni exists at the level of the digestive tract, the liver and in all the tissues of the body. In the digestive tract it exists as acid in the stomach; enzymes in secretions from the mouth, stomach, small intestine and pancreas; and as bile from the liver. It also refers to the mixing functions of the stomach and intestines, the reabsorption of water and salts in the large intestine, as well as the process of eliminating the stool from the body.

The digestive process can be profoundly affected by our state of mind and what is happening for us emotionally. Who hasn't experienced a loss of appetite or butterflies in the stomach prior to a public-speaking engagement or an important exam? Emotional stress affects the wave-like contraction of involuntary muscle in the digestive tract that propels food towards the anus. Disruption of this process can produce symptoms such as bloating, abdominal distension, constipation and diarrhoea.

From an Ayurvedic perspective, the role of the mind and our emotions on the functioning of our digestion and thus on our physical health is a given. Western medicine also acknowledges the role of stress in digestive disorders such as irritable bowel syndrome and ulcerative colitis. The direct link between the mind and the gut has also been explored in the work of Gerda Boyesen, the founder of a school of body-oriented psychotherapy based in London.

While working as a physiotherapist in psychiatric hospitals in Oslo, Norway, she noticed that while she was massaging her patients she would frequently hear digestive gurgles coming from their abdomens. She then decided to investigate further and placed a stethoscope on the abdomens of her patients while she was massaging them. Using this approach she started to discern recognisable patterns of sounds that correlated with relaxation taking place in their bodies as a result of her massage. As the patients relaxed deeply, tension held in their visceral organs would be released, producing gurgling sounds.

The wave-like contraction of involuntary muscle in the wall of the bowel is known as peristalsis. Realising the direct connection between our mental and emotional state and the movement of food along the bowel, she coined the term psycho-peristalsis.

Health tip

A cup of warm water with a squeeze of lemon juice first thing in the morning is an excellent way to stimulate a satisfying bowel movement.

As a yoga teacher myself, I have frequently noticed the amount of audible tummy rumbling at the end of the yoga class when patients are lying down on their backs in the corpse pose. Having released a lot of tension held in their bodies during the class they are able to relax deeply, so the gurgling begins! Unfortunately some of my students are very embarrassed at the sound of their digestive tracts, so I point out that this is a normal part of the relaxation response and a very natural phenomenon.

The different digestive capacities of the three body types

Ayurveda, with its appreciation of body type, recognises that the digestive fire is different in people with different body types. The three basic body types are held to have different digestive tendencies. People with more Vata in their nature have an irregular digestion, and their appetite is changeable – sometimes it is very strong, at other times non-existent. They can forget to eat and become spacey when they miss a meal. In the past they would have been labelled as having a sensitive stomach. They do well with smaller and more frequent meals in general. Children with more Vata in their nature tend to have an indifferent relationship with food, much to their parents' annoyance, and tend to be pickers.

People with more Pitta in their nature have a regular, strong appetite and are unlikely to ever miss a meal. If the meal is late coming to them they can become irritable and fiery. They need three square meals a day in order to feel satisfied. As children they have a tendency to bolt down their food and can easily overeat, sometimes getting a reputation as garbage-guts.

> THE KEY TO BETTER MANAGING YOUR DIGESTION IS TO LISTEN TO YOUR BODY.

People with more Kapha in their nature have a steady appetite. They like to graze throughout the day and don't worry too much if they miss a meal or if it's late. They have a tendency to comfort eat, which can result in weight gain. Children with more Kapha in their nature are particularly drawn to dairy products and will often have food stashed away in their bedroom and pockets.

Once you have a sense of where you fit in relation to your type of agni, you can then start to better manage your digestion and the functioning of your immune system. The key to better managing your digestion is to listen to your body. As your awareness becomes more refined, you will begin to notice what eating habits serve you best.

In my medical practice, I find that some patients have already worked out for themselves, through a process of trial and error, what approach to eating is best for them. More often than not, the approach that they have worked out for themselves is in accord with what I would recommend for them based on my understanding of their Ayurvedic body type. So the empirically derived approach of the patient is affirmed by the theory of Ayurveda – a nice meeting place between patient and practitioner.

Honouring your agni

The timing, the environment and the manner of eating are given a lot of attention in Ayurveda. At this point I would like to explore these themes further, with the proviso that these are only general guidelines and each individual will need to fine-tune them for themselves using their intuition.

Many of our current approaches to eating in the West are very limiting and are definitely not in our long-term health interests. The experience of one of my students, in this regard, is salutary. Vicki, a 25-year-old IT worker, has worked for the same corporation in London, Sydney and Bangkok. The eating cultures in London and Sydney were very similar – lunch is generally eaten, somewhat apologetically, in front of the computer screen. However, in Bangkok, the approach was entirely different. At midday all work would stop on the floor and the IT workers would go down one floor to a communal cooking and eating area. The food would be prepared, the woks turned on, and then the freshly cooked meal served to the workers. Then at 1 pm, with the kitchens cleaned, everyone would return to their workstation on the floor above. This communal style of sharing food together has long been a part of Thai culture for good reason, and the social benefits are most apparent. At a time when corporations are looking at ways of improving morale and goodwill in their staff, this must surely be a most simple and expedient approach.

Health tip

As your agni is strongest in the middle of the day, this is the best time to have your main meal.

The Industrial Revolution has certainly had a significant influence on our eating habits. In most traditional cultures, lunch was the main meal. As transport was limited, most people would eat their lunch at home and then return to their workplace – at their shop or in the fields. At the end of the day, they would return home, probably tired after a full day, and take a light evening meal before retiring to bed. As our digestion is strongest in the middle of the day, this is the natural time to have our most substantial meal. Also we have the rest of the day to digest the food as we walk around and tend to our business.

Nowadays, more often than not we travel away to work, using public transport or our cars, and return at the end of a long day to our homes. As we have worked hard, it is only natural to want to have some kind of reward for our labours, which tends to come in the form of a hearty dinner. Dinner finished, we may well then want to relax in front of the TV, before retiring to bed. From an Ayurvedic perspective, this is a recipe for overwhelming the agni and for indigestion. Not a lot of digestion takes place once we are horizontal or asleep, so this kind of lifestyle encourages weight gain and the build-up of ama in our bodies.

A holistic approach to managing your agni

As well as attending to the kind of food and drinks we consume and how we consume them, Ayurveda recognises that in order to balance our agni we need to take a holistic approach. What does this mean in practice? Essentially it means that we need to be supporting and nurturing ourselves in various ways – including working with the body, the mind and emotions and with the spiritual dimension of life. These themes will be explored in some detail in later chapters of this book. At this point, I would like to outline what I mean by a holistic approach; an approach that embraces the physical, emotional, mental and spiritual levels of our being.

Embracing the physical, emotional, mental and spiritual

The physical level refers to the three traditional pillars of healthy living – food, exercise and sleep. The quality and quantity, as well as the timing, of the food and drink we consume have a clear impact on our agni. Regular, preferably daily, exercise appropriate for our age and our level of fitness supports the agni. Good quality sleep and adequate rest helps to rejuvenate our internal fire and prevents burnout. I would also include supplements, such as herbs, vitamins and minerals, as additional ways of supporting the agni.

The emotional level, in my experience, is the least supported level in most people in the West. Many of us have been influenced by a post-war culture of getting on with life where our emotional needs have not been honoured. Our basic need to have our feelings validated and acknowledged, rather than overlooked and dismissed, has not been met during our formative years. The resulting emotional disconnection and suppression adversely affects the agni, and can create health imbalances and disease.

Having a loving partner, friends and family is certainly a great help in supporting the emotional level. But there may be issues that we find hard to talk about with them or which we would prefer not to burden the relationship with. It also happens that the people we are most intimate with may have some kind of agenda, which makes it hard for us to be completely open with them. For these reasons, I have become an advocate of what I call proactive psychotherapy, where you deliberately choose to involve a health-care professional to provide an additional layer of psychological support.

A useful definition of psychotherapy, taken from *Introduction to Psychotherapy* by Dennis Brown and Jonathan Pedder, is as follows: 'A conversation which involves listening to and talking with those in trouble with the aim of helping them understand and resolve their predicament.' In proactive psychotherapy there does not need to be any specific 'trouble'; the person may be interested in having a more loving relationship with a partner or relative, they may want to understand themselves better or develop their communication skills.

Health tip

Developing skills in emotional literacy is a powerful way to support your agni.

Dylan, a client of mine in his late forties, decided at my suggestion to engage the services of a psychotherapist to help him repair his relationship with his only daughter, Chloe. His wife had died suddenly several years earlier and his relationship with Chloe had become distant and at times frosty. His efforts to get closer to his daughter had met with very limited success and he was at a loss as to what to do next. Needless to say, the situation was causing him a lot of emotional pain and was very confusing to him. I referred him to an older female psychotherapist to help him see things from a woman's perspective and to enable him to better understand Chloe. Happily, through working with the psychotherapist, Dylan was able to open up a more meaningful dialogue with his daughter and begin to heal the rift in their relationship.

Psychotherapy aims to create a supportive environment where you feel able to talk freely and to allow yourself to connect with your emotions. It's a place to explore your thoughts, feelings and behaviour with a view to solving problems and living a happier, healthier and productive life. It is dependent on building up a trusting relationship with your psychotherapist; a relationship that has the benefit of being confidential and professional in its nature.

Counselling and psychotherapy can help you develop skills in emotional literacy. By this I mean the ability to recognise, understand and appropriately express your feelings and emotions. It also helps you to empathise with other people and to work through experiences that could be potentially emotionally damaging. These skills are essential in negotiating your needs in significant relationships and in resolving interpersonal conflict.

It is important that the therapist is well trained and experienced and it helps a lot if they come to you recommended by someone whose judgement you trust. It is also desirable if the therapist has some degree of natural wisdom about them and that you feel intuitively comfortable in their presence. If the therapist has done a considerable amount of work on themselves through their own psychotherapy and spiritual practices, this will help create a much more egalitarian feel to the way in which you work together.

IT IS OFTEN EASIER FOR OTHER PEOPLE TO SEE HOW THESE ATTITUDES AFFECT OUR BEHAVIOUR ...

The mental level relates to unconscious beliefs or attitudes that we hold and which drive our behaviour and actions. It is often easier for other people to see how these attitudes affect our behaviour than it is for us to see them in ourselves. Most of us know someone with a chip on his or her shoulder, but the person in question doesn't usually know that. More than likely they have a story about life that they are emotionally invested in, and which prevents them from seeing other points of view. Perhaps they believe that men can never be trusted or that people will always try to take advantage of you if you let them. Needless to say, such belief systems are very limiting and can prevent us from living to our full potential. They can also do tremendous harm to our most important relationships. When self-esteem is low, it is difficult for individuals to feel worthy of being loved and this can result in a lot of suffering for them.

Working to heal these deeply held attitudes can be helped by good psychotherapy; psychotherapy that is affirming and supportive in nature and which allows trust to be built up slowly over time. It is also true that being part of a supportive community can be very important in facilitating healing. In a modern context this may come through various kinds of groups in which we feel safe to express ourselves authentically and where we can be among like-minded people. Twelve-step programs, personal development seminars, men's groups and religious fellowships, to name only a few, can be very helpful.

The spiritual level relates to coming to terms with such basic questions as: 'Who am I? What will happen to me when I die? And where was I before I was born?' This is necessarily a highly individual process and an ongoing enquiry as we journey through life. It is an area that a lot of people find very challenging and where satisfaction is lacking. From time to time, I also see patients who have a very rich spiritual life including a cherished daily spiritual practice, a practice they draw a great deal of nourishment from and which sustains them through each day. (I return to this subject and examine it in some detail using the lens of some of the ancient spiritual traditions of India in Chapter 8.)

While managing your digestive fire is an holistic process, it is certainly true that simple changes to your eating habits can go a long way to improving your overall health and sense of wellbeing.

 ## Managing my digestive fire

Anjani, an Ayurvedic colleague of mine, healed digestive problems that had plagued her throughout most of her life using an approach inspired by Ayurveda and yoga.

After a fourteen-year career as a corporate lawyer in top-tier law firms in both the UK and Australia, I had become very ill and depleted. I was chronically anxious and suffered from severe sleeping problems and panic attacks. I had no energy and was emotionally frail and physically exhausted. But that was not the worst of my problems. I suffered from chronic food intolerances.

My food intolerances had begun many years earlier, with severe stomach bloating after eating bread. This persisted and became gradually worse over a period of about nineteen years until it became chronic. I was unable to eat wheat, gluten, garlic, chilli, dairy, tomatoes, all fruit, and most vegetables. Eventually all I was able to digest safely was boiled chicken and rice, and even this was sometimes problematic.

If I did eat any other foods I would experience severe stomach bloating and pain, and this often led to severe bouts of diahorrea and vomiting. I would experience heaviness and sleepiness after meals. I was admitted to hospital on many occasions due to the chronic pain, which would sometimes be so severe that I would pass out.

Western medicine diagnosed me with IBS (irritable bowel syndrome), but could not treat it. I tried many alternative therapies including acupuncture, naturopathy and Chinese medicine. You name it, I tried it, but to no avail. In my attempts to find an alternative remedy, I was introduced to the science of Ayurveda.

After only four months of studying Ayurveda, I cured myself of all my food allergies. I can now eat everything, even gluten, garlic and chilies. I did this simply by using the right herbs, food and exercise routines for my own unique doshic body type.

What I discovered was that I had been suffering from a lack of digestive fire. As someone with a lot of space and air elements in my body type, the main qualities of my body–mind are cold and dry with not much fire. My work as a lawyer, and even my intensive studies to become a lawyer, demanded a lot of fire. You can say that law is a fire job. So not having a naturally strong digestive fire, and then requiring lots of fire to study and then work as a lawyer, essentially put out my digestive fire. As a result, my digestion was unable to cook the food I was putting into my body.

To remedy this, I began to literally stoke my digestive fire. This was done similarly to if you were to make a fire outside with wood. This entailed eating warm, moist foods with the opposite qualities to the cold, dry qualities of my body type. My diet also consisted of cooked foods rather than raw food. This helped to lighten the load on my digestion until I could get the fire burning again. I used warming herbs with my food to help cook the food as I ingested it. These included black pepper, cinnamon, turmeric, cumin, ginger, asafoetida, nutmeg and cloves. I would drink warm herbal teas instead of cold drinks and sip all liquids, not gulp, to avoid putting out my digestive fire. My largest meal is always taken at lunchtime when I'm most active and my digestive fire is naturally highest. My evening meal is usually a very light soup or broth.

Getting a good sweat going is crucial to stoking the digestive fire. Once you are sweating, you know that the body is metabolising. So wearing lots of layers of clothing and engaging in exercise helps stoke the digestive fire. I found that once I got a sweat up (the layers of clothes help do this quickly), I only needed 15–20 minutes of exercise four or five times per week to keep my fire stoked.

Finally, adopting an eating ritual helped me the most. It is of vital importance to do nothing while eating. The simple act of sitting quietly at a table, focusing only on eating, chewing each mouthful well, relaxing the stomach and the mind are all fabulous ways to help boost the digestion and eliminate food intolerances for good.

Some simple Ayurvedic suggestions for improving digestion

Avoid eating a heavy evening meal. Ayurveda advocates making lunch our main meal when our digestive fire is at its strongest. Once we go to sleep our digestion slows down markedly and it is difficult for food to get properly broken down and assimilated. When this happens we are more likely to feel heavy and lethargic in the morning and have no appetite. Unfortunately in our post-industrial revolution society, having the main meal in the evening is the norm. As a result a lot of people are slow starters in the morning and require coffee to get them going.

Eat only when you are hungry. While this may seem like common sense, it is certainly true that we often eat for other reasons – out of habit, because of the time of day or because we are feeling bored or anxious about something. This extra food places a load on our digestion and interferes with our natural appetite for food.

Avoid cold drinks and eating food straight from the refrigerator. Your body temperature is 37 degrees Celsius, so iced drinks and cold food will douse the digestive fire and make it harder for the body to warm up, break down, absorb and assimilate food.

Sip fluids during the meal as dictated by your intuition. If you imagine the stomach as one of those portable cement mixers seen at building sites, you can better understand how some fluid at mealtimes helps the food to mix. How much fluid feels right will depend on a number of factors including the nature of the food, the hydration status of the person eating and their body type. In general terms people with more Vata in their nature do well having ample fluid with their food; people with more Kapha in their nature need less fluid; and people with more Pitta in their nature are somewhere in the middle. What amount of fluid feels right is necessarily highly individual and will change from one meal to the next. Here, your intuition is your best guide.

Silence or light relaxed conversation is desirable at mealtimes. Many people are sensitive to the emotional tone at the table when they are eating and find it hard to eat if there is conflict in the air. The practice in some families of resolving conflict

> **Health tip**
>
> For most people, the easiest way to improve your general health and immune system functioning is to have a light evening meal.

at the dinner table is a recipe for digestive upset. So the general recommendation in Ayurveda is to eat when you are eating, rather than combining it with reading, watching television or being on the computer. It is then that a meal can be a truly nourishing experience.

Try not to eat heavily when feeling very emotional. There is a tendency in some people to stuff down their emotions by eating a lot of food. While this is understandable, it does impair the digestive process. Ayurveda therefore suggests eating lightly when you are highly emotional, whether with anger, grief or anxiety. Drinking a herbal tea, such as peppermint or chamomile, can be a useful substitute to a meal and helps to settle your digestion and nervous system.

Chew your food well. In the words of Mahatma Gandhi, 'Chew your drink and drink your food.' Essentially this means taking time to draw nourishment from your food and drink, enjoying the process of chewing the food and the taste of it in your mouth and on your tongue. Avoid gulping down your fluids but allow the taste to be experienced fully in the mouth, almost like a wine taster.

Eat around the same time each day. Your body likes routine and naturally likes to be nourished at similar times each day. It gets confused if one day breakfast is at 6.30 am, the next day at 9 am and the next day at 8 am. While this is not something to be applied rigidly, it does help if you can aim to eat at roughly the same time each day for breakfast, lunch and dinner.

Take a short walk after your evening meal. Rather than plopping down onto the couch and watching TV, consider going for a walk or sharing doing the dishes with the people you live with. Ayurvedic texts recommend a walk of one hundred paces on the flat. The erect posture helps the movement of food along the digestive tract and activities such as walking or doing the dishes can be an important time for conversation and catching up with significant people in your life.

Hara haichi bu – eating to 80 per cent of your capacity

Hara haichi bu is an established dietary practice among the Okinawan people who live on the small islands in the southernmost prefecture of Japan. They are famous for being one of the healthiest and most long-lived people on the planet. In many Okinawan communities, it is common to find people living active and independent lives who are well over one hundred years old. Hara haichi bu involves only eating to 80 per cent of your stomach's capacity, thereby allowing space for the proper mixing of food and ensuring a comfortable digestive process. The Ayurvedic approach is very much in agreement and suggests that at the completion of a meal your stomach should contain one half solid food, one quarter liquid and one quarter space.

Overeating is very common the world over and creates various kinds of indigestion from heartburn and bloating to abdominal colic and excessive wind. For many people, overeating is a habit not easily broken. By being consciously aware of the food in front of you, the people you are eating with and how you are feeling when you sit down for a meal, you will be less likely to overeat. Closing your eyes and taking some slow relaxed breaths is a good start and helps you to feel more connected to yourself and your environment.

Fasting to strengthen the digestive fire

Fasting is known in Ayurveda as langhana because it creates lightness in the body-mind. It is another way to help build up the digestive fire, particularly when it has been overwhelmed by excessive food consumption and lack of exercise. Fasting needs to be appropriate for your Ayurvedic body type, as intense or prolonged fasts can actually aggravate Vata dosha and deplete the body's energy reserves.

When approaching the task of creating a fast for yourself, it is also important to take into account what kind of foods feel intuitively right for you. During the fast it is very helpful to drink warm water or herbal tea throughout the day. I include here some simple fasts that can be used with different body types and help to restore the digestive fire to a balanced state.

Three-day fasts

Vata-dominant individuals

Breakfast: Stewed fruit (such as apples and pears) with ¼ teaspoon of cinnamon powder

45

Lunch: Khichari (this is a risotto-like dish suitable for all doshas made from rice, lentils and vegetables that is mildly spiced and very easy to digest, see recipe page 74)
Dinner: Pumpkin, carrot or vegetable soup

Pitta-dominant individuals
Breakfast: Fresh fruit salad
Lunch: Khichari for all doshas (see recipe page 74)
Dinner: Green vegetarian salad

Kapha-dominant individuals
Breakfast: Stewed fruit (such as apples and pears) with ¼ teaspoon of cinnamon and ¼ teaspoon of clove powder
Lunch: Khichari for all doshas (see recipe page 74)
Dinner: Spicy vegetable soup or herbal tea

Herbs and spices to strengthen the digestive fire

Kitchen herbs and spices such as cumin, mustard, ginger, turmeric, fennel, black pepper, fenugreek and curry leaf, are routinely used in Ayurveda to kindle the digestive fire. As many people today have a weak digestive fire due to a sedentary lifestyle and poor dietary habits, incorporating herbs and spices into your diet can be extremely helpful in strengthening the agni.

Herbs and spices can be used in the cooking process, taken before meals or enjoyed as a meal accompaniment in the form of fermented pickles or chutneys. Chewing on a small slice of fresh ginger coated in sea salt and sprinkled with lime-juice fifteen minutes before a meal is a traditional home remedy to stimulate the appetite and strengthen the agni.

The herbs and spices encourage the gentle movement of food along the digestive tract and help make the food more digestible. Some herbs such as black pepper also help burn up ama or toxins in the digestive tract. I explore the use of kitchen herbs and spices in the promotion of good health in more depth in Chapter 10.

Chapter 4

Eating well, feeling well

Let food be your medicine.

Hippocrates

Most of us have experienced a meal, the memory of which endures for decades. It may have been a fish barbequed over a small fire in a distant Asian country, a romantic dinner with your partner at a restaurant with a fabulous view and immaculate service, or a home-cooked Christmas lunch with your extended family. Usually, there is a combination of factors that have come together to leave a lasting impression. The freshness of the ingredients, the loving intention of the cook, the physical setting and the good company you shared the meal with are all important parts of the mix.

When it comes to meals that stick in my own memory, I am immediately cast back to a small Indian village in the foothills of the Himalayas. It was 1987 and I was working as a volunteer doctor in a small hospital run by the Tibetan government in exile in Dharamsala. One of the Indian teachers at the local Tibetan Children's Village had invited me for dinner at his home.

It was a cool November evening and the aromas of cumin and basmati rice were already wafting through the house when I first arrived. The sound of stew bubbling on the fire could be heard as we sat and chatted before the meal.

I still remember how the teacher's wife adeptly managed the simple wood-fire stove made from moulded clay. The stove was complete with two hot air vents that ran from the central hearth and kept the various pots of food warm. She had prepared rajmah for us, a subtly spiced kidney bean stew, and carefully served us while we sat around the fire to ward off the chill of the mountain air.

The meal was washed down with a draft of fresh water from the family well, then by way of a digestive, we went for a relaxed walk at sunset through the corn and winter paddy fields that surrounded the village. We then returned home for a cup of masala chai, a sweet, milky tea spiced with cardamom and ginger.

There was a purity about the whole experience that impressed itself indelibly on my mind at a time when my interest in food and cooking had not yet surfaced in my life. From an Ayurvedic perspective all the necessary requirements were met for a truly nourishing meal. My five senses had been stimulated. I was relaxed, in good company, and fully receptive to the food that had been lovingly prepared. The choice of ingredients and the way they were prepared were ideal for the early winter season. Not surprisingly the experience of the meal created a contentment that lasted long after I had finished eating.

... THE EXPERIENCE OF BEING NOURISHED IS MUCH MORE THAN THE PHYSICAL ACT OF CONSUMING THE RIGHT MIX OF CARBOHYDRATES, FATS AND PROTEINS.

For many people living a busy modern lifestyle, meals are seen as a time to put petrol back in the tank in order to give you energy to get through the day. By contrast, the experience of being nourished is much more than the physical act of consuming the right mix of carbohydrates, fats and proteins. Nourishment is a more complex phenomenon and could best be described as an energetic experience that sustains us physically, emotionally, mentally and even spiritually. Put simply, it is the difference between a home-cooked meal shared with friends in relaxed surroundings and eating takeaway in front of our computer at work.

In this chapter I introduce some of the essential principles of the Ayurvedic approach to nourishment; an approach that encourages us to enjoy our food to the maximum and at the same time to use it to balance our body, mind and emotions. Whether eating alone or sharing food with our family or friends, meal times are seen as one of the most sacred of our daily rituals.

Ingredients

One of my students, a confirmed India-phile, shared her experience of the best lassi she has ever tasted. Lassi, for the uninitiated, is a drink made from yoghurt and water popular in the subcontinent. It can be sweet or salty in flavour and helps digestion if taken towards to the end of a meal. Sweet lassi has fruit added to it. The yoghurt, water and fruit are mixed together using a blender, often with a pinch of cardamom powder added.

While staying in Goa, she came across a roadside stall that just sold one thing – strawberry lassi. The lassis were so good that each afternoon a crowd of people would gather around the stall to get their lassi. After enjoying these sweet, creamy offerings for several consecutive days, she finally asked the vendor, 'What's your secret? What makes these lassis so good?' The man then beckoned her to follow him and they walked straight through his family home and emerged into his back garden, where he presented to her his much loved cow – Lakshmi.

Health tip

Adding home-grown herbs is a simple way to enrich the quality of your food.

In Ayurveda, the relationship between the grower and the food is fundamental to understanding the qualities of the ingredients. Has the food been grown on a farm practising mono-agriculture, where one or two crops are raised on large tracts of land and where the agricultural practices can only be sustained through the use of herbicides and insecticides? Or has the food been grown on a certified organic farm practising biodiversity and utilising sustainable methods?

As consumers, we can bring a considerable degree of influence to bear on the food industry by the way we spend our dollars. Our choices in the marketplace can determine whether a product will sink or swim in the supermarket shelves. When I first started teaching Ayurvedic cooking classes in the early 1990s in Sydney, there were only a few health food shops that stocked organic milk. Twenty years later, both the leading supermarkets chains now stock their own brands of organic milk.

Ayurveda encourages us to have a more intimate relationship with the food we consume. As such, growing our own vegetables and herbs allows us to be closer and more involved in the self-nourishing process. It may be as simple as growing some oregano and basil in a pot on the balcony of your flat or participating in a community garden. Some may be fortunate enough to have their own veggie patch that can be fertilised with composted material from their kitchen.

Food that is organically grown, fresh off the farm or from the back garden, tends to have an inherently greater life force than food that comes from large-scale farms using an industrial approach. By contrast food that has been in storage for months to years tends to deteriorate quickly when left out in the open in the kitchen fruit bowl.

Ayurveda favours fruit and vegetables grown locally. This food will be more appropriate as it will reflect the season and climate you are living in. As a medical student living in Ireland, I would venture down to the local supermarket to buy the food for our student house. As we had limited means, I soon became aware of what were the cheapest items in the supermarket. Not surprisingly, I ended up buying vegetables in season – onions, potatoes, turnips, brussels sprouts and cabbage. Given that it was winter in a temperate climate, these kinds of vegetables were wholly appropriate and became staples in our diet.

When food is processed, its vital force is diminished. If we take the example of sugar and flour, we get an idea of the extent to which food processing has become an integral part of our food culture. White sugar and white flour are both highly refined food products, far removed from sugar cane and whole grains of wheat. From an Ayurvedic perspective, it is better to go with less processed forms of sugar such as jaggary or rapadura sugar, which are essentially dried sugar cane juice, and to use wholegrain organic flour.

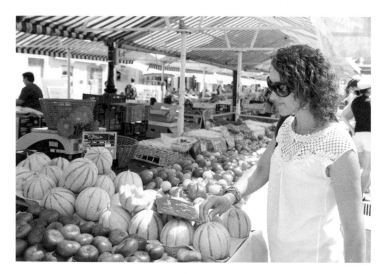

Food as energy

Ayurveda sees food as energy that can restore balance to your body–mind or make you feel out of balance and potentially create disturbances to your digestion. It understands the energy of food through its qualities. Is the food warm or cold, light or heavy, moist or dry, rough or smooth, oily or non-oily? Foods that are considered to be heavy and harder to digest include meat, wheat pasta, legumes, dairy products and oily foods, such as foods that have been deep-fried. Light foods are easy to digest and include stewed fruits, soups, consumes and steamed vegetables. Moist foods include casseroles, wet curries, soups and dahls, whereas examples of dry food include dried fruit, biscuits, corn chips and rice crackers.

The beauty of this approach is that you can appreciate the energetic qualities of different foods for yourself by simply tuning into your five senses. You can then use this understanding to see what kinds of foods are most likely to balance you.

Using the principle that like increases like, Ayurveda enables you to know how food is likely to affect you.

> USING THE PRINCIPLE THAT LIKE INCREASES LIKE, AYURVEDA ENABLES YOU TO KNOW HOW FOOD IS LIKELY TO AFFECT YOU.

For example, if someone with more Vata dosha in their nature consumes a lot of cold, dry food and iced drinks, their Vata dosha will increase. If they continue to do so over the next few weeks, their Vata dosha is likely to get aggravated. This may well result in symptoms of abdominal upset with bloating, gas and constipation, and feeling spacey, scattered and agitated.

If a person with more Pitta in their nature consumes a lot of hot spicy food, their Pitta dosha will increase. If they make a habit of doing this, then over time their Pitta dosha is likely to become aggravated. This might result in heartburn, stomach acidity, outbursts of anger, irritability and the appearance of skin rashes. If someone with more Kapha dosha in their nature consumes a lot of cold, heavy stodgy food their Kapha dosha is likely to increase. If they continue this habit, this might result in weight gain, sinus congestion, lethargy and low mood.

Another way that Ayurveda understands the energy of food is through its taste. Six tastes are traditionally described – sweet, sour, salty, pungent, bitter and astringent – all having different effects on our physiology. The sweet taste includes foods such as most vegetables and fruits, and cereals such as rice and wheat and milk. The sour taste is found in citrus fruits, tamarind, vinegar and yoghurt;

the salty taste is present in salted foods, soy sauce, tamari and pickled foods. The pungent taste refers to foods that are hot and spicy in nature such as garlic, onion, ginger, pepper and other hot spices. The bitter taste is the one that is most often avoided and is found in bitter melon, dandelion, coffee and the bitter lettuces like radicchio, endive and chicory. Finally the astringent taste is one which causes a puckering of the palate and has a drying effect on the body. It is found as a secondary taste in some fruits and vegetables including slightly unripe banana, pomegranate, cranberry and black tea.

The six tastes in foods

Sweet taste	most fruits, vegetables, rice, wheat, milk
Sour taste	citrus fruits, vinegar, yoghurt
Salty	soy sauce, olives, tamari, salted foods
Pungent	most spices including ginger, garlic, pepper, onion, mustard seed, chilli
Bitter	radicchio, endive, dandelion, coffee, fenugreek, turmeric, bitter melon
Astringent	unripe banana, pomegranate, black tea, cranberry, peanut butter

Each of the six tastes has a specific effect on the human body-mind. The sweet taste has a cooling effect on the digestive process and is essentially nourishing, promoting the growth of the body's tissues. It is said to give contentment when taken in moderation, but in excess it can create obesity and sluggishness. The sour taste has a mildly warming effect on the body-mind and helps to kindle our digestive fire (agni). It is said to awaken the mind and dispel intestinal gas. When used in excess it can create a souring of attitude and irritation.

The salty taste is used in Ayurveda to stimulate the appetite, particularly when a small amount is taken before a meal. The salty taste is moistening and grounding and has a mildly warming effect on the body. It draws water into the tissues of the body. As such, it is beneficial for Vata body types that are prone to dehydration, but in Kapha body types it can cause fluid retention.

The pungent taste is the hottest of the tastes, it promotes tears and nasal secretions, purifies food and is said to give clarity to the mind. In excess the pungent taste has a weakening effect on the body and can induce weight loss.

The bitter taste is light, dry and cold in its qualities and has a cooling effect on the body-mind. It is the taste most often lacking in the Western diet and is said to restore the sense of taste. The bitter taste promotes the digestion of toxins and is sometimes taken after meals in India. Mahatma Gandhi was in the habit of chewing on neem leaves, which are very bitter, on finishing his meals. Used in excess the bitter taste has a depleting effect on the body and causes wasting of the body's tissues. In Ayurveda the bitter taste is described as the most spiritual taste because, like suffering, most people try to avoid it.

The astringent taste is dry, light and slightly cooling and has a contracting effect on the tissues of the body. It promotes the absorption of fluids and is useful in treating diarrhoea. In excess it can create constipation, dryness of the mouth and weakened vitality.

Ayurveda encourages us to include all six tastes in each meal in order to make it truly balanced. If this is not possible, it recommends having all six tastes present in at least one meal each day.

Using food to balance your body, mind and emotions

Rather than making generalisations about what food is good or bad for you, Ayurveda, above all, asks the question, 'Who is the food for?' It encourages you to be mindful of your body type and how you are feeling when choosing your food and drink. Are you an office worker with a sedentary lifestyle or a young man in his twenties working on a building site? The Ayurvedic approach is always oriented to the individual and his or her unique set of dietary needs. The food that may best suit a woman with a Kapha-dominant body type struggling to keep her weight down will be very different to the kind of food best suited to a woman with a Vata dominant body type who is losing weight. It encourages you not to take a one-size-fits-all approach but to find a diet that will be appropriate for your body type, lifestyle and any health imbalances you may have.

In order to keep yourself balanced, Ayurveda uses the Law of Opposites. Essentially this means balancing the qualities in your bodily experience using food with the opposite qualities. For example, if you are feeling cold, warm food is advocated; if feeling heavy, light food is recommended. If you are feeling scattered and spacey, heavier, grounding foods are best.

In this simple process, you first need to tap into your bodily experience. You can do this by closing your eyes, connecting with your body through breathing consciously, and then asking yourself the question, 'How do I feel? Physically? Emotionally? Mentally?' You then wait and see what answer, if any, comes to you.

- If you're feeling cold and dry, perhaps a little anxious, go for food that is warming, cooked, mildly spiced and moist, such as soups, dahls and casseroles with adequate amounts of good quality salt. This will help to keep you warm and grounded.

- If you're feeling hot and dry, perhaps irritated or frustrated, eat food that is cold in temperature, cooling in nature and moist, such as salads, fresh juice blends, cold soups or a cold mixed vegetable tart; foods that keep us calm and cool.

- If you're feeling cold and heavy, perhaps lethargic, stuck or gloomy, beneficial foods are warming, well spiced, dry and light, such as stir fries and dry curries; foods that are stimulating in their nature.

- If you're feeling depleted physically and emotionally, favour light, easy-to-digest foods such as soups, especially made with root vegetables and spiced with digestive spices like cumin, coriander, turmeric and curry leaf. Foods that will help you feel well nourished.

- If you're feeling like you're on an emotional rollercoaster, favour a light diet and consider missing a meal and replacing it with a herbal tea or light soup instead. Eat a more substantial meal when feeling less emotionally provoked. Sucking on a few cardamom seeds or having a warming herbal tea such as ginger can often be helpful. You lighten the load on your digestion in these ways.

Approaching food and drink in this way adds another dimension to your relationship with food and in my experience serves to enhance your enjoyment of food. The basic principles outlined above become a starting point for your own personal approach to the selection, preparation and consumption of food. It's an approach that uses your intuitive faculty to fine-tune what you really feel like eating. It also opens up the possibility of using food medicinally when you are feeling unwell and proactively attending to your health at the first sign of malaise.

Several years ago during a three-day bush walk in the Budawang mountains south of Sydney, I had cause to make use of my Ayurvedic awareness around food.

It was mid-winter and snow had fallen on the day prior to the beginning of our walk. An icy 50-kilometre wind was blowing. Staying warm, even given the strenuous nature of the walking, was challenging. Our first night was spent sheltering in a large overhang cave, aptly named the Tiltin' Hilton, as the floor of the cave was sloping. After a sleepless night, not helped by the uneven surface and the howling wind, I woke feeling dreadful.

Lying there in my sleeping bag, I knew that I needed warmth and nourishment to face the day. Happily my brother-in-law was already up, having slept better than I had, and had a small campfire going. I asked him to make me a cup of tea with extra sugar (I normally take no sugar), which he kindly brought to me in my sleeping bag. I then spent the next ten minutes savouring the hot liquid with every morsel of awareness I could muster, feeling it move through my digestive tract bringing my body back into balance. The results were amazing. At the end of that cup of tea I felt as if I had moved from feeling a lowly 20 per cent to a reasonable 80 per cent. My muscles felt less tight, my nervous system was soothed and my mood lifted!

Eating in line with your Ayurvedic body type

As well as tapping into how we are feeling from moment to moment, we also need to be mindful of our Ayurvedic body type in how we approach food and drink. I include below some general principles regarding diet that can be a useful guide to balancing your body type.

The Vata body type

People with more Vata dosha in their constitution do best with food that is warming, easy to digest and grounding. They do well with food that is cooked, adequately spiced and salted and moist in nature. They are advised to favour food that is sweet, sour and salty in taste. The sweet taste is the most nourishing taste and helps to build up tissue; the sour taste is warming in its effect on the body; and foods that are salty in taste help the body to retain fluid, as salt attracts water. For these reasons soups, casseroles and wet curries are excellent for balancing Vata dosha.

Eating regularly and at set times is an important key to managing Vata dosha, as missing meals tends to aggravate Vata. Many people with a Vata-dominant body type cannot tolerate too much raw food because it is harder to digest and can often produce wind and bloating. Sipping warm water throughout the meal is a good practice for individuals with a Vata dominant constitution.

The Pitta body type

People with more Pitta dosha in their constitution do best with food that is cooling, and require a reasonably substantial meal in order to feel satisfied. As they have a strong appetite they need to watch for a tendency to overeat. They do well with raw food that is bland in nature. However, they are very attracted to hot, spicy food that only causes them to overheat.

Pitta types are advised to favour food that is sweet, bitter and astringent. The sweet, bitter and astringent tastes are all cooling in nature, and the latter two are also drying, thereby balancing the moistness of Pitta dosha. For these reasons salads, leafy greens, bitter foods and most fruits are important staples for balancing Pitta dosha. Sipping room temperature water throughout the meal is generally recommended for individuals with more Pitta in their nature.

The Kapha body type

People with more Kapha dosha in their constitution do best with food that is light, dry and spicy. They are prone to comfort eating and need to be careful with too much snacking. Consuming heavy, stodgy food will aggravate their tendency to sluggish digestion, as will overeating. They are advised to favour foods that are pungent, bitter and astringent in taste. Pungent food is warming and stimulating in its nature and is ideal for Kapha dosha. Bitter and astringent tastes are both drying and therefore counterbalance the moistness of Kapha.

People with more Kapha in their nature do well with dry curries, stir-fries and mixed steamed vegetables. Sipping warm water or ginger herbal tea throughout a meal is very balancing for them.

Foods for the doshas

Vata-pacifying diet: favour foods that are sweet, sour and salty

Fruits	Sweet, ripe and juicy; warm stewed fruit is best in winter; avoid dried fruits, which are wind-forming
Vegetables	Most vegetables are balancing to Vata, especially if well cooked; raw vegetables and vegetables such as cabbage, brussels sprouts and cauliflower can be wind-forming; good to favour root vegetables
Grains	All rice including brown rice, wheat, oats (cooked)
Legumes	Red lentils and yellow mung dahl
Animal foods	Free-range chicken, eggs, seafood, beef occasionally
Dairy	All dairy products are okay in moderation
Nuts	Most nuts are okay in moderation
Seeds	Sunflower, pumpkin, sesame, flax and chia help to pacify Vata dosha
Spices	Cumin, mustard seed, fenugreek, asafoetida, cinnamon, cardamom, ginger, turmeric, sea salt, black pepper in small amounts
Oils	Sesame, olive, ghee, coconut

Pitta-pacifying diet: favour foods that are sweet, bitter and astringent

Fruits	Most fruits are balancing to Pitta with the exception of sour fruits such as citrus
Vegetables	Most vegetables are balancing to Pitta with the exception of raw onion, shallots and tomato; leafy greens are most favourable.
Grains	Rice (basmati), wheat, oats (cooked), barley
Legumes	Yellow mung dahl, soybean products such as tofu and adzuki beans are recommended
Animal foods	Free-range chicken, egg white, freshwater fish
Dairy	Unsalted butter, cottage cheese, ghee, cow's milk
Nuts	Soaked almonds and coconut; most nuts being oily can aggravate pitta dosha
Seeds	Sunflower, psyllium pacify Pitta dosha; pumpkin in moderation is okay
Spices	Coriander (leaves, seeds and powder), fennel, mint, turmeric, saffron, cardamom, cumin and small amounts of fresh ginger
Oils	Ghee, olive, coconut and sunflower

Kapha-pacifying diet: favour foods that are pungent, bitter and astringent

Fruits	Pomegranate, cranberry, figs, raisins, apples, papaya, pears, grapes
Vegetables	Light vegetables such as leafy greens, asparagus, potato, cabbage, cauliflower, brussels sprouts, eggplant, okra, capsicum
Grains	Barley, buckwheat, corn, millet, rice, quinoa
Legumes	Most are well tolerated, though too much tofu can disturb their digestion
Animal foods	Free-range chicken, eggs, fish
Dairy	A low dairy diet is recommended, goats milk, diluted yoghurt
Nuts	Nuts being oily tend to aggravate Kapha dosha
Seeds	Chia; flax, pumpkin and sunflower are okay in moderation
Spices	All spices, including chilli in moderation.
Oils	Safflower, mustard and light olive oil

For a more detailed examination of the principles of Ayurvedic nutrition and cooking I recommend *The Ayurvedic Cookbook* by Amadea Morningstar. This book includes extensive information on how different foods and dishes affect the three doshas and includes plenty of simple recipes that are not overly time consuming to prepare.

Bi-doshic body types

People with fairly equal amounts of two doshas in their body type need to be mindful of both their doshas when it comes to food selection. It is helpful if they tune into how they are feeling and the state of their doshas before preparing and eating their food. For example, if you identify yourself as having a Kapha–Vata body type and are feeling heavy and sluggish, you would do well to favour a Kapha-pacifying diet. By the same token, if you are feeling anxious and dehydrated, you would favour a Vata-pacifying diet.

It is also important to be aware of the season in determining what foods are likely to be most balancing for you. For someone with a Pitta–Vata body type, a Pitta-pacifying diet is most appropriate during the warmer months of summer and spring, and a Vata-pacifying diet is most appropriate during the cooler months of autumn and winter. Use these principles as general guidelines, letting your intuition have the last say.

Food selection

When shopping at the greengrocer or fruit and vegetable section of your local supermarket, bringing your intuition to bear on the process of food selection while being mindful of your body type and the season, will go a long way to making sure your nutritional needs are well met. As described previously, I recommend closing your eyes, centring yourself with a few deep breaths and then asking yourself the question, 'What do I really feel like eating at this time?'

At this point, rather than engaging your intellect, wait for the answer to come to you. It will often appear to you in precise detail; for example, I feel like having corn on the cob, with some melted butter and some cracked pepper. You will soon know if you have accurately tuned into your intuition by how you feel when eating the meal and afterwards.

Eating ethically

One of the guiding principles of yoga, Ayurveda's sister science, is ahimsa or non-violence in how we think, speak and act; a principle wholeheartedly embraced and made popular by Mahatma Gandhi during his lifetime. An aspect of ahimsa relates to the choices we make about the kind of food we eat and by extension the food industries we choose to support or not.

In the case of eating the flesh of animals, it involves making an assessment of the quality of life of the animal as well as how it was slaughtered. Was it raised and treated in a humane way during its lifetime?

Most pigs spend their entire lives raised indoors in pens of concrete and steel and increasingly cattle are fattened up in feeding lots prior to slaughter. On lots of levels, these conditions are inherently stressful for the animals. Chickens, unless they are certified free range, are housed in small cages in factories where they are unable to move about and experience stress from unnatural levels of overcrowding.

Factory farms also produce large amounts of urine and faeces that end up in large cesspools that have at times overflowed into nearby rivers killing millions of fish and destroying river eco-systems.

When considering eating fish and seafood, it is important to look at the kind of fishing practices involved. Many of these fundamentally deplete the world's fish and seafood stocks and sometimes involve scooping the seabed floor, creating untold damage and destruction to sensitive marine eco-systems. Fish factory ships are becoming more common. It is estimated that one-quarter of all fish caught each year are by-catch: fish that are not wanted and are thrown overboard dead or dying.

Health tip

Next time you buy coffee, check if it has fair trade certification.

If we choose to consume milk and dairy products, it is worth considering the life of the dairy cow. In modern dairy farming, mother cows are separated from their calves at an early age creating acute grief for the mother cow. As dairy cows are made to produce milk continuously throughout their lives, this causes considerable stress on their bodies and they are generally slaughtered well before their natural life span of 20 years.

In response to these ethical concerns, some people will choose to become vegans, not consuming animal products of any kind. Others may choose to become ovo-lacto vegetarians and support farmers who have strict ethical codes around the treatment of dairy cattle and chickens. Some may choose to include fish in their diet that is caught by companies using sustainable approaches, and eat only certified free-range chicken. There are many possibilities in terms of finding an approach that sits comfortably with your core values.

Another aspect of eating ethically is buying coffee, tea, chocolate and other products that involve fair-trade agreements with small farmers in developing countries. Traders seeking fair-trade certification are required to pay a price to farmers that will cover the cost of sustainable production, which they can live on and that allows them to invest in development.

By choosing to buy organic produce, we can help reduce the use of harmful pesticides and herbicides that enter into soil and water systems and which can adversely affect the health of farm workers and farmers living in close proximity to farms using such products. Avoiding genetically modified food sources is another important way that we can try to eat more ethically.

Ultimately we all have to make a decision about where we stand in relation to the ethics surounding the food we choose to consume. For anyone interested in exploring this important subject in more depth, I recommend the book *The Ethics of What We Eat* by Peter Singer and Jim Mason.

Conscious cooking

Ayurveda encourages you to bring an intentional awareness to the process of food preparation. This begins with the sourcing of the ingredients for the meal and continues right through to the moment that you serve food. When approached with the right attitude, this can be an extremely satisfying endeavour that benefits the whole household and is nourishing on many levels.

Making sure that you have a clean and uncluttered space in the kitchen is an important start and sets the tone for the ensuing process. Once that is established, it helps if you can take some time to mentally connect with the person or people you are cooking for. If you are cooking for your family, getting another family member involved in the process of washing and chopping vegetables saves time and allows you to share the task. It also means that some of that person's energy will be in the meal and helps them to feel more connected to the food and the creative process of cooking.

As someone who does a lot of cerebral work in my chosen vocation as a healthcare practitioner and teacher during the day, I find it very grounding to work with my hands at the end of the day. The practical process of cooking helps to get me out of my head and distances me from my work, providing an important time of transition.

Cooking is an essentially sensual experience. Ayurveda encourages you to tune into all of your senses when preparing a meal – how the food sounds, smells, feels and looks. The sizzle of mustard and cumin seeds in a saucepan of hot sesame oil, the aromas that fill the kitchen, the luscious feel of hand-mixing a mango and rocket salad and the feast of colours when you stir-fry red capsicum, snow peas and yellow squash – these are all to be enjoyed and savoured.

> AYURVEDA ENCOURAGES YOU TO TUNE INTO ALL OF YOUR SENSES WHEN PREPARING A MEAL ...

As Ayurvedic cooking encourages the use of spices, I include here a useful guide to spicing a dish, and suggest how you might consciously approach the cooking and serving of a meal. First, heat your preferred oil or ghee in a frying pan and then add whole seeds such as mustard or cumin, and later fresh spices such as ginger or garlic. These spices will flavour the oil. At this point chopped vegetables are added and mixed well so that the oil can coat the vegetables. Next sprinkle the more delicate spice powders such as turmeric or coriander over the vegetables and add leafy spices such as curry leaf and coriander to the mix. Then add the required amount of liquid and again mix well with a wooden spoon. Most often the liquid will be coconut milk although whey and water are also used in some recipes.

At this stage, after further stirring, the frying pan can be covered and the food can continue to cook on a lower heat. As this is a less intensive stage in the creative process, it is a good time to organise setting the table and let other members of the household know that dinner is not far away.

Once the food is cooked, it is a good practice to turn off the heat and allow it to settle. The next five to ten minutes are an important transition time as you move from the intensity and activity of the creative process to being in a more relaxed and receptive state to enjoy the food. Without this interval, it is very difficult for the cook to really be present for the eating of the meal and regain his or her appetite. How often do you hear the cook of a delicious meal say apologetically that they have no appetite!

With the cooking done, I recommend that cooks wash their hands, move out of the kitchen and sit quietly to allow themselves time to settle; they can then call the rest of the household to the table and serve the food or, preferably, get someone else to serve the food!

Mealtimes

I once heard a Franciscan monk make the point that Christ spent a lot of time with his followers coming together over meals in a spirit of communion, as immortalised in the painting *The Last Supper*. Certainly there are few things more sustaining in life than sharing a delicious meal with family or friends in a warm, relaxed environment.

The conscious inclusion of small rituals at mealtimes can go a long way to create an atmosphere that encourages connection and camaraderie. I include here a number of simple suggestions to help you be more present to the experience of nourishing yourself with food.

Firstly, when your plate is in front of you, a useful practice is to close your eyes and consciously tune into your whole body by being mindful of your breath. Secondly, I suggest closing your eyes and consciously smelling the aromas of the food in front of you. This act, in itself, can be deeply nourishing, though it is surprising how few people tune into their sense of smell before a meal. Next, when your eyes have opened, consciously appreciate the colours of the meal in front of you. This is particularly important to people with more Pitta dosha in their nature, who tend to have a strong visual orientation.

If eating with others, taking a few moments to connect with the people you are sharing the meal with and to inwardly honour them, and their presence in your life, is another way to nourish yourself. You may also choose to verbally acknowledge the cook of the meal at this juncture. Many cooks are underappreciated, so this small act can go a long way to lifting their spirits after all their labour.

Saying some form of grace or a statement of gratitude for the nourishment that the universe has provided for you is another way of enriching the meal experience. While this is a very individual matter, a ritual of some kind can bring in another level of awareness for the eaters and imbues the meal with a sense of togetherness. One friend of mine makes a point of verbally acknowledging all the people involved in bringing the food to the table, from the grower right through to the cook.

I include here a simple grace without any specific religious overtones that was passed on to me. It comes from a woman named Sandy.

We honour ourselves and each other
By taking the time to be here.
This food is a gift and a blessing;
It nourishes our bodies and souls.
We cherish
these times
together.

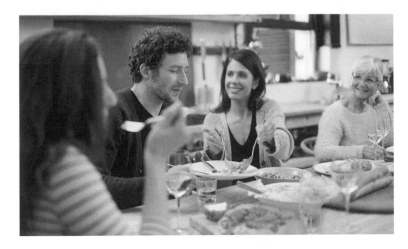

Tips for families

Most families have a spread of different body types. This need not be a problem for the cook as there are a number of simple ways to cater for individuals with different doshic make-ups. From the outset, it is important to say that food that is made from fresh ingredients, which is mildly spiced and salted and cooked with love, tends to be balancing to all three doshas.

Someone with more Vata in their nature will generally want a smaller helping and additional salt with their meal. Ayurveda recommends using good quality sea, lake or rock salt. They also tend to like dishes that have plenty of sauce in order to feel satisfied. Someone with more Pitta in their nature will want a larger helping and may require plenty of raw food, while a person with more Kapha in their nature will enjoy adding pungent spices such as black pepper or chilli to their food. This can be facilitated with a shaker of chilli powder or some spicy chutney.

A small spicing skillet can be a great investment for the family and allows spices to be added to the already cooked food just prior to serving. By sautéing spices such as mustard seeds, cumin seeds, fresh ginger or garlic in some ghee or vegetable oil you can make a spice combination known as a tarka or chaunce. This can then be mixed into the food by those who prefer spice.

... THIS MEANS TURNING OFF THE TELEVISION, RADIO AND OTHER COMPUTER SCREENS WELL BEFORE THE MEAL STARTS.

It is the responsibility of the parents in the family to set the tone of the culture around mealtimes. In practical terms, this means turning off the television, radio and other computer screens well before the meal starts. It is helpful and practical to get children involved in the process of preparing the meal, even if only in a small way. This can be achieved by getting them to chop vegetables, find ingredients in the cupboard or set the table. In this way the meal is something they have contributed towards, rather than something that has magically appeared on the table at the appointed time!

Parents can also initiate conversations at mealtimes that talk about the food – where it came from, the ingredients, how it was cooked and whether people at the table like it or not. This can lead into discussions about the day just passed, things that were fun and things that were not so good. While this kind of interaction can be harder to get going with teenagers, once established in a family it can have a life of its own.

At the end of the meal, the process of clearing the table, looking after the washing of dishes and tidying the kitchen can also be an important time of household communion. As well as fulfilling a practical need, it allows you to spend time with your family in a shared space working with a common intent. At the end of the process there is the satisfaction of having completed a task together. It also encourages children to take responsibility around the home. In our house, the cook is always exempt from doing the washing up, which seems only fair!

Food combining

Ayurveda holds that certain food combinations disturb the normal functioning of the digestive fire, or agni, producing toxins known as ama. In Ayurvedic cooking you try to skillfully combine the qualities of the foods to make them easier to digest and enhance their absorption and assimilation. For example, you might add a pinch of ginger or cinnamon to lighten a heavy food like oatmeal porridge or bring to the boil a cold food like milk to make it more digestible.

Most vegetables are relatively easy to digest and can be readily combined with other foods in meals. Cooking a vegetable makes it lighter and more digestible. Adding herbs and spices that enhance digestion, such as cumin, turmeric, coriander and ginger, will further support the process of digestion.

Fruits tend to be slightly oily and will promote digestion if eaten early in the meal or before it. Similarly, salads tend to produce a lot of gas and flatulence when taken at the end of a meal. There are also certain foods that combine well, such as tomatoes and basil, and cooking legumes such as kidney beans and lentils with spices such as cumin and turmeric. These principles are recognised in many different culinary traditions around the world.

Cooking for my family the Ayurvedic way

Robyn, a 59-year-old holistic counsellor, shares her approach to cooking for her family with their different body types and health needs.

Ayurveda has become an integral part of my life since 1996 when I first went to India. I undertook studies in Ayurvedic lifestyle counselling some years later as I wanted to share this wonderful knowledge with my family.

I began by introducing Ayurvedic cooking principles. What I discovered with Ayurveda is that even small changes can make huge differences. Being the cook in the household, food was a way to try and keep our doshas balanced and our digestive fires healthy.

The cooking aspect took some consideration, as although we varied only slightly with our body types, there were minor health issues and personal likes and dislikes. My husband is predominantly Pitta with Vata secondary and could not tolerate very spicy foods nor oily foods as he has had his gall bladder removed. I am predominantly Vata with Pitta secondary and required warming spices and oils in my cooking, especially during the cool, dryer months of the year. My daughter is Pitta–Vata and loves spicy foods, especially chilli, and she also suffers from asthma, which is worse during winter. My stepdaughter is Vata–Pitta and can suffer from Kapha imbalances in winter connected to her love of dairy-based foods.

The starting point was to find the overlap for all our doshas and then work from there. At the same time I wanted to honour the effects of the seasons on our bodies and minds regardless of our dosha type. I decided to include all six tastes in preparing our meals and be mindful of varying environmental and emotional conditions as well as the individual's body type.

To address these factors I use naturally sweet foods as they are beneficial for both Pitta and Vata. I avoid very pungent spices and fried foods all year round since they aggravate Pitta and are too drying or hard to digest for Vata. I emphasise warm, moist and nourishing foods mildly spiced with warming spices in autumn and mid-winter to pacify Vata dosha.

When it is cold and wet both my daughters suffer from congestion so I add mildly drying herbs and ground pepper to balance their Kapha dosha. I also reduce heavy foods such as dairy products. In the hot season I favour cooling and lighter foods to pacify Pitta dosha. As my husband can only tolerate small amounts of oil and spice, I add more heating spices cooked in ghee in a separate pot for my daughters and myself halfway through the cooking process.

During winter we usually sit down to an organic grain breakfast of rice or oats that has been well cooked in milk with freshly grated ginger, nutmeg and cinnamon. Alternatively, we

> have fruits such as seasonal local apples stewed with mildly warming spices including clove, nutmeg and cinnamon and at the end I add a drizzle of ghee for my daughters and myself.
>
> During summer I sweeten our breakfast with dry-roasted coconut and a little maple syrup for a cooling quality. As an alternative to porridge we may have organic spelt toast or a homemade chapatti with a spread of avocado and a squeeze of lime juice. We also enjoy seasonal fresh, sweet, soft organic fruit such as mangos, coconut, fresh figs, dark grapes and sweet melons for breakfast or as a snack.
>
> For the main meals, although I cook a variety of assorted vegetarian meals, I favour dhals and vegetable dishes. My favourite legume is split mung bean as it balances all three doshas and is easy to digest.

Food cravings

During my training in obstetrics and gynaecology as a medical student, I undertook a study of pica in pregnancy. Pica is the medical term for food cravings that are sometimes experienced by pregnant women and children. I found that 25 per cent of the women I interviewed experienced some kind of unusual food craving. Sometimes the cravings were for relatively common foods such as pickled onions, but in researching the topic I came across a case where a pregnant mother-to-be had a strong urge to suck on pieces of coal. Presumably some part of her organism knew that she needed something in the coal to support a healthy pregnancy.

Ayurveda recognises two different types of cravings. The first type of craving is held to be biologically driven and is designed to bring the organism back into a state of balance. In my medical practice, I have come across a pregnant mother, herself a strict vegan, who was having powerful cravings for steak. She was in a quandary, not wanting to go against her heartfelt philosophical commitment to veganism, but keen to do the right thing by her unborn child. As it turned out, she did go ahead and eat some red meat and though she did not enjoy the experience, her energy levels and vitality improved dramatically within days of her carnivorous dalliance. She reported feeling better in herself than she had in months.

While food cravings may be more apparent in pregnant women and children, Ayurveda holds that we all experience food cravings throughout each day. The fact that many people do not register these cravings tends to be a product of our culture and conditioning here in the West. As we have previously noted, many people are not connected to their intuition and do not trust it. It is also true that when we are stressed or caught up in a busy lifestyle, we are often less receptive to the quiet voice of our intuition.

The second type of craving is more commonly experienced and is driven by emotional needs and habits. Chocolate, salty foods such as potato crisps, and sweet foods such as cakes and biscuits are favourites. In order to differentiate these two types of cravings, you need to simply pay close attention to how you feel during and after consuming the food. When the craving is in line with your intuition, you tend to feel satisfied at a deep level; your body says 'yes' unequivocally.

When you are in a state of relative balance, you tend to be attracted to foods that will support balance in your body–mind. Your bodily intelligence is speaking clearly to you and is reflected in the kind of food and drink you are naturally attracted to. When you are out of balance, you will be attracted to food and drink that will take you further out of balance. In general, individuals whose Vata dosha is out of balance will go for cold, dry and light food, such as rice crackers, corn chips and biscuits. Those individuals whose Pitta dosha is out of balance will go for hot, spicy foods such as chilli-laden stir-fries and curries. This kind of food is particularly appealing to them as it causes them to perspire and cool down. However, in the longer term the chilli has a warming effect and can result in overheating. Individuals whose Kapha dosha is out of balance will go for sweet, heavy foods such as cheese, yoghurt, ice-cream and cakes.

 Going with my gut

Following your intuition is not always an easy thing to do, especially when you are experiencing different types of cravings. JL, a 25-year-old university student, shares how Ayurveda has been useful in working with his intuition.

I began learning about Ayurveda a few years ago. I remember being introduced to it as the science of intuition. I liked that definition. It intrigued me.

My studies of Ayurveda explored doshic imbalances. My new insight was that when a dosha is out of balance an action that feels right will generally be an action that further exacerbates the imbalance.

A common problem I had was with Vata dosha – I was often feeling spaced out, exhausted and disconnected. At these times I noticed that listening to my intuition seemed to suggest more meditating, eating lighter foods or fasting and contacting friends who I know are also Vata types. What shocked me when I looked at this was that it wasn't just a random selection of actions that I was intuiting was right for me, it was the exact actions that would make my imbalance worse, and often did.

Now when I have an intuition of what to do I first check if I feel balanced or imbalanced. If I'm imbalanced I think the action through in terms of how it might affect my doshas. Often I find it's not just unhelpful it's actually the exact thing NOT to do. Then I just have to think of the doshic opposite and go with that until I feel back in balance.

Kitchen alchemy

Why is it that food cooked with love and eaten in the home of friends or family is so much more satisfying than food served in fine restaurants? There seems to be an X-factor in operation that is unmistakeable. It's as if the food is imbued with a subtle quality; a quality that we can feel, although it would be difficult to measure using modern scientific methods. In Ayurveda, this special quality of food is known as the prabhava. It refers to the hidden power of a food. It's a power that we can all experience and that can lift a meal from being simply tasty to being one you will remember for the rest of your life, right down to the minutest detail.

For eighteen years I ran Ayurvedic cooking classes in Sydney with my friend Tim Mitchell. Out of the hundreds of dishes we cooked during those years only a few really stand out; there was something about them that had that WOW factor and which everyone in the class could appreciate. One in particular was a Sri Lankan eggplant curry that I demonstrated how to make. Once the basic ingredients had been brought together in the frying pan, including coconut oil, an array of spices, organic eggplant and coconut milk, the dish then required careful stirring. When

I asked for a volunteer, a woman who identified herself as having more Kapha dosha in her constitution immediately shot up her hand. Excited to be doing something active, she came up to the cooking bench and gently stirred the pot for the next 30 minutes, while we prepared some other dishes.

As we have seen previously, individuals with Kapha dosha in their make-up tend to have a nurturing disposition and are generally blessed with plenty of patience. Happily for us all, she took to her job with great devotion and lovingly applied herself to the task of stirring the dish. Not surprisingly, the eggplant curry was by far the best dish of the many we cooked that day and was loudly praised by all the cooking class participants.

Naturally good cooking is an art form. An art that requires knowing your ingredients and understanding how to combine them to bring out flavour and texture. It requires an intimate knowledge of your stove and cooking utensils as well an appreciation of how long to cook things for and how to use herbs and spices to bring a meal alive. That said, the attention the cook gives to the process of cooking is of paramount importance. As we all know, a few distracted moments answering a telephone call can have a disastrous effect on the final product.

When we are really present to the cooking process and tuned into our five senses, we are more able to make the subtle changes required to bring out the best in a meal. This tends to occur when we love the whole experience of cooking and are strongly motivated to produce a beautiful meal. My friend Martin, who runs a popular vegetarian café in Darwin, is endowed with a naturally nurturing disposition. He describes being at his happiest when preparing healthy and delicious meals for his customers, many of whom he knows well. It is almost as if he is cooking for his extended family and he talks about entering the zone when busy making quiches, Bali curries, papaya salads and coffees for his customers. (See page 201 for Martin's quinoa treat.)

My experience of the Ayurvedic approach to nutrition

I include here an account written by an old student and friend of mine who works as an IT consultant. She describes how she approaches nourishing her family – an approach to cooking and nutrition that has been taken up by her teenage son.

I had followed a strict yogic vegetarian diet for fifteen years, but in that time, had often suffered from significant tummy cramps and lower digestive tract issues. After I moved away from the regimented yogic diet, I found the Ayurvedic principles of nourishing yourself. I differentiate a diet as a prescribed course of eating, whereas the Ayurvedic principles are essentially an understanding of how to nurture your health.

Practising Ayurveda is about establishing those good habits that sustain you. As you practise Ayurveda and develop a healthy respect for your own needs, you also naturally develop a healthy respect for individual differences and personal needs. As a mother this helped me to respect what my children needed and hopefully in doing so, helped them do the same for themselves, so that they may respect their own physical needs and nurture themselves with that consideration.

Ayurveda has a wonderful approach to digestion that considers and celebrates eating on all levels – colours, aromas, textures and flavours. This also means that food is naturally enjoyed and shared with gratitude, and so nourishes the soul as much as the body.

What Ayurveda does for us most powerfully, is to consider and celebrate who we are as we enjoy our food. My husband's favourite food is and always will be the food that his mum cooks. As a mother, I wanted to establish for my children fond and nourishing memories of food. One of the things we did was to celebrate Thanksgiving with our dearest friends enjoying and sharing wonderful food.

Practising Ayurvedic principles can take many forms. For example, we experience very fast-paced lives, and so every Friday, at the end of the working week, my son purposely creates a slow-cooked stew. It takes about four hours to cook and is the best meal of the week. I can see him with his children one day throwing an array of meat, vegies and herbs into a cauldron, enjoying the aroma wafting through the home while patiently waiting to enjoy a delicious feast in which they savour the fruits of taking things slowly and gently.

Eating out

Ayurveda extols the benefits of eating food you have cooked yourself or that has been cooked by someone that loves you. When eating out it is preferable if you have some kind of connection with the chef and cooks. For these reasons I prefer to eat at family restaurants where I have an established relationship with the cooks and the staff waiting on the tables. While this is not always possible, it is certainly a criteria worth considering when thinking about dining out.

Ayurvedic cooking is often thought to equate with Indian cooking, but this is inaccurate. It is simply using the principles of Ayurveda when preparing food. At our Ayurvedic cooking classes, we have prepared food from a variety of different cuisines including Italian, Middle Eastern, Indonesian, Moroccan and Russian dishes.

In general, people with more Vata in their nature do well with soups, dahls and moist saucy foods that have been well cooked. It is usually possible to find something on most menus that is pacifying to Vata dosha. They need to beware of dry foods such as corn chips, cold foods such as ice-cream and eating too much raw food. People with Pitta-dominant body types do well with most types of salads and raw foods. Blessed with strong stomachs they can tolerate a wide variety of cuisines, but need to avoid garlic-laden Mediterranean foods, oily takeaway food and Asian dishes laced with chilli. People with Kapha-dominant body types do well with dry, light and spicy food, such as Asian dishes low in oil found in Thailand, Korea and south India. They need to avoid heavy, creamy foods more common in northern European cuisines. A light stir-fry or dry curry is ideal.

The beauty of the Ayurvedic approach is that you will always be able to find a dish right for you on any given menu, by being mindful of the state of your doshas and what your intuition is telling you.

Health tip

When eating out, be mindful of the vibe in the kitchen, as this will permeate the food you are eating.

The Ayurvedic approach to alcohol

As with other aspects of our diet and lifestyle, Ayurveda recommends a moderate and conscious approach to drinking alcohol. The stimulating and dulling effects of alcohol on the mind and nervous system were well understood by the ancients and drinking alcohol was not favoured for people interested in meditation and spiritual life. It is also true that Ayurveda uses medicated herbal wines, known as arishtams, to promote healing, especially when the digestive fire is low. A small amount – around 60 ml – of herbal wine is prescribed and taken at mealtimes.

In a modern context, it is important to be aware of how alcohol affects you physically and mentally, and to be mindful of your body type when choosing your alcoholic beverage. Individuals with more Vata dosha in their nature need to be careful with cold, iced and bubbly drinks such as beer and sparkling wines that can potentially aggravate Vata dosha. These type of drinks depress the digestive fire and can lead to excessive gas, bloating and abdominal discomfort. Warm or room-temperature drinks are therefore preferable and non-sparkling wine is better tolerated than beer.

Individuals with more Pitta in their nature are better able to tolerate beer, especially in summer, as they tend to a have strong stomachs. However, the heating effect of alcohol on the body can aggravate Pitta dosha causing heartburn, hot flushes and aggression in the short term. Wine, fortified wine and spirits, which have a higher alcoholic content, are particularly aggravating to Pitta dosha and in the long term create heat in the body, especially in the liver.

People with more Kapha dosha in their nature can feel invigorated by the stimulating effects of alcohol; however, as alcohol is also a depressant, it can also cause them to feel lethargic and flat if taken in excess. As Kapha dosha is cold in nature, room temperature or warm drinks, such as mulled wine, are preferable.

The diuretic effect of alcohol, which causes the body to become dehydrated, can also aggravate Vata dosha in everyone, so keeping your water intake up when having a drink is recommended. While alcohol may initially make people feel more relaxed, as the body withdraws from alcohol, it can make some people, especially more sensitive Vata-dominant individuals, feel anxious and cause sleep disturbances.

Two meals that are balancing for all three doshas

It is certainly possible to cook food that is nourishing and appropriate for all three body types and balances all three doshas. Here are a couple of recipes that can be used in this way. They are quick and easy to prepare and can be adjusted for the season and for taste.

Khichari

This is a classic Ayurvedic dish. It is particularly easy to digest and is used to restore digestive health. This recipe was demonstrated to me by an Ayurvedic colleague who makes large pots of it a couple of times a week and then home delivers servings to his friends and clients. Khichari is profoundly nourishing and can be used all year round. Feel free to experiment with different herbs and spices, using your intuition as your guide.

½ cup basmati rice

½ cup split mung dahl

1 tablespoon ghee or olive oil

1 pinch asafoetida (also known as hing, available from Indian grocery shops)

1–2 teaspoons mustard seeds

1–2 teaspoons cumin seeds

1 teaspoon fenugreek seeds

1 bay leaf or 5 curry leaves

1 teaspoon coriander powder

1 teaspoon turmeric powder

3 cm (1¼ inch) ginger, grated

8 cups water

vegetables, chopped into 2 cm (¾ inch) cubes (eg pumpkin, zucchini, spinach, beans)

Celtic sea salt to taste

1 lemon, juiced

more water, as required

yoghurt and finely chopped coriander, to serve

- Thoroughly wash rice and mung dahl.
- In a large saucepan (or pressure cooker) warm ghee and then add asafoetida, mustard and cumin seeds. Cook until mustard seeds begin to pop and turn grey and cumin seeds turn a darker brown colour. Add fenugreek seeds towards the end of this process and cook until a darker shade of brown. Make sure not to overcook fenugreek seeds, as they can become very bitter and dominate the dish.
- Add the leaves, coriander, turmeric powders, ginger and then add rice and mung dahl. Mix well so the ghee coats the grains. Add water and continue to stir, bringing the mixture to a boil. Simmer for about 45 minutes over medium heat.
- Add vegetables and cook for another 15–20 minutes. Add salt towards the end of this process. Add lemon juice to the khichari and mix well.
- Turn off heat, cover and allow to slowly cool. To serve, garnish with a dollop of yoghurt and coriander.

Seasonal mixed vegetables

This is a versatile vegetable and grain combination that can be modified for body type, season and intuitive preference. It was developed at the Ayurvedic cooking classes I taught with Tim Mitchell over many years in Sydney.

2 teaspoons ghee or olive oil

1 pinch asafoetida

1–2 teaspoons brown mustard seeds

1–2 teaspoons cumin seeds

1 onion, chopped

2 cm (¾ inch) ginger, grated

vegetables in season:

    1 whole sweet potato, cut into cubes, and 1 cup of peas; or

    2 large carrots, sliced and 1 handful of green beans; or

    2 large zucchinis and ½ a butternut pumpkin, cut into cubes; or

    ½ a cabbage, coarsely chopped and 1 whole corn, kernels cut from the cob

1 teaspoon turmeric powder

1 teaspoon coriander powder

5–10 curry leaves (fresh, if possible)
150 ml (5 fluid oz) water or coconut milk (optional)
Celtic sea salt and black pepper to taste
1 bunch fresh coriander or continental parsley coarsely chopped
basmati rice, to serve

- Heat the ghee in a medium-sized saucepan over moderate heat and when hot, add a pinch of asafoetida, which will form into tiny bubbles when the oil is hot enough. Next add the mustard seeds and when they begin to pop, add the cumin seeds and heat until they go a darker shade of brown.
- Add the chopped onion and sauté for a few minutes and then add the ginger to sauté for a few more minutes before adding the chopped root vegetable, spice powders and curry leaves.
- Mix the ingredients together well and then add some water (or coconut milk, if desired) until the tops of the vegetables are covered. Once the root vegetable is three-quarters cooked, add the other vegetable (peas, zucchini, etc.) and cook until tender.
- Towards the end of the cooking process add sea salt, pepper and most of the coriander or parsley. Mix well and cook for a few more minutes. Cover the saucepan with a lid, turn off the heat and let the food settle for 5 minutes.
- The consistency of the mixture can be varied according to taste, but ideally should be slightly liquid and not too thick and stodgy.
- Serve on a bed of freshly cooked basmati rice (or you may like to experiment with other grains such as quinoa, millet or couscous). Garnish with a little more coriander and/or parsley and enjoy!

Accompaniments for both dishes – depending on season, body type and intuition
- Yoghurt spiced with a little cumin powder and sea salt
- Buttermilk
- Mango or other fruit chutney
- Pappadams
- Chapatti or roti (flat, unleavened bread)
- Fermented pickles

Chapter 5

Honouring your body

Your body is the temple of the Holy Ghost.

I Corinthians

The sister sciences of Ayurveda and yoga both acknowledge that your body is wise. It is not just the flesh and bones that carry around your brain, but a highly intelligent part of you, which has intimate connections with your mind. By contrast, the Western philosophical tradition has tended to separate the mind and the body. Rene Descartes, the 17th century French philosopher who is credited with a well-known version of this view, argued that the mind and the body were distinct substances. The human mind and intellect were seen as god-like, and the body as the seat of animal passions and sexuality. It was our link with the animal kingdom and something that needed to be tamed in order for the human race to move forward. As human beings we were set apart from nature and this has had far-reaching consequences in terms of how we relate to our bodies.

Certainly the cultural orientation in the West has been intent on rising above the needs and demands of the body rather than one of validating and acknowledging them. The 'no pain, no gain' principle has held sway in large measure and produced an attitude to the body dominated by suppression. In this context it is quite normal to ignore or quash bodily symptoms rather than listen to them and do what you can to honour them. In India and other ancient traditions, we find a very different way of relating to our bodies – an approach that acknowledges the fundamental connection between body, mind and spirit.

How yoga sees the human being

In the tradition of yoga, the human being is conceived as having five sheaths, much like the layers of an onion. These sheaths are generated as consciousness descends into denser and denser matter.

Each sheath provides a platform for the expression of consciousness at that level. Subtler sheaths act as templates for the grosser sheaths, with each level of organisation building on the previous one.

The five sheaths are called koshas in Sanskrit and are energetically connected to each other. Each sheath has a particular function in the body–mind–spirit complex.

1. Anna-maya-kosha: Literally 'the sheath composed of food'; is the most gross sheath. It is nourished by the juices extracted from our food and corresponds to the physical body.

2. Prana-maya-kosha: Literally 'the sheath composed of life force'. This body connects the sheaths of food and mind and is nourished by prana. Prana is our life force and will be better known to some readers as qi, the equivalent term in traditional Chinese medicine. Our prana is an energy that is replenished in two main ways: from breathing air and from digesting food in the gut. It animates the physical body.

3. Mano-maya-kosha: Literally the 'sheath composed of mind'; corresponds to the mental body and is nourished by words, images and emotions. It is dominated by the activities of the small mind; the chatter of thoughts that accompany us throughout our daily activities.

4. Vijnana-maya-kosha: Literally 'the sheath composed of wisdom'; corresponds to the psychic body and relates to our core values and our capacity to reason and make judgements.

5. Ananda-maya-kosha: Literally 'the sheath composed of bliss'; is closest to our essential nature. It holds our deepest joy and peace and functions as a silent witness to our lives, unmoved by all our emotional ups and downs and dramas.

The five sheaths of the human being

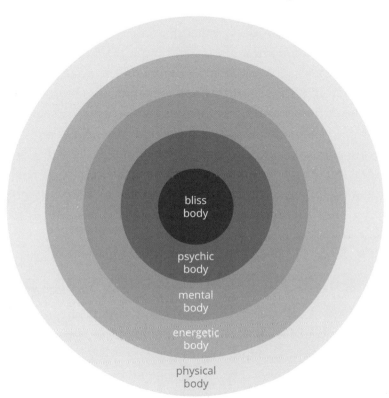

There is an intelligence that exists in all these layers. Essentially we are seen as an energetic whole – a complex interplay between the spirit, the mind and emotions, and the physical body. Some writers have coined the term 'the cosmic computer', which gives us an idea of the complexity of this matrix. This being the case, our body becomes a much-cherished resource that is speaking to us all the time, not a nuisance that must be overcome in order for us to get back to our activities at work, at home or on the sports field.

In the present age, when we're so infatuated with technology, it's hardly surprising that we have become more disconnected from our bodies and what they are trying to tell us. We are quite happy to feed our intellects all sorts of ideas and theories, but our bodies come a poor second. We have lost touch with our bodies and the richness of their experience and accordingly they have shut down in the face of such neglect. No longer understanding the language of our own bodies, we are forced to run to various types of healthcare professionals to fix the problem.

It is also true that yoga in the West in large part has come to mean the practice of yoga postures and has been incorporated into our gym culture. Here the focus is on physical exercises that promote fitness and make the body look better. Looking good has become a major subtext in the culture of some yoga schools, catering to our society's obsession with physical attractiveness rather than inner harmony and beauty.

Both yoga and Ayurveda encourage us to cultivate a more conscious relationship with our body. Using various yoga postures, breathing exercises and other self-care practices we are able to rekindle a more loving connection with our bodies and ourselves in ways that help us to feel more relaxed, grounded and content. In this chapter I would like to address how you can do that using simple practices that can be incorporated into your daily routine.

Cultivating a simple home practice of yoga postures

Most of us accept that in order to prevent the build-up of plaque on our teeth, it is necessary to brush our teeth each day, preferably two or three times, in order to reduce the possibility of cavities and developing holes in our teeth. For most people, brushing and/or flossing are an accepted part of their daily routine. The yogic paradigm holds that we build up physical, emotional and mental tension through the process of living and that it is important for our long-term health and wellbeing to release this tension on a daily basis. If allowed to accumulate, this tension can result in chronic musculoskeletal problems, mood disturbances and physical illness, as well as a reduced enthusiasm for life.

Regular exercise is certainly helpful in reducing different forms of stress and anxiety and builds up strength in the body. Most people will attest to its utility in promoting a sense of vitality and in keeping you feeling more buoyant in mood. This process can be further enhanced by cultivating a practice of yoga stretches or tai chi that can be done at home. These ancient practices have the added benefit of promoting suppleness in the joints and relaxation in the muscles, something that is not often achieved through simple exercise.

In addition, they promote what is known as body–mind integration. What do I mean by this? Body–mind integration practices foster a more harmonious connection between your thoughts, your mood and what is going on in your physical body. By combining bodily movement, awareness and our breath, you enter into a very different relationship with your body. We can also use these practices to release tension held in the body and develop a better understanding of how the mind and emotions affect the functioning of our bodies.

After 15–20 minutes of these practices, most people feel lighter in their bodies and more relaxed, and have a greater sense of personal wellbeing. With ongoing practice and the supervision of a good teacher, you develop a greater capacity to enter into the simplicity of the here and now, rather than being caught up in the incessant ramblings of your mind.

With so many people becoming time poor in the 21st century, establishing a short home practice of yoga postures makes a lot of sense. As yoga is an oral tradition, it is preferable to approach a yoga teacher who you respect and arrange a one-on-one class with them. The aim of this class would be to put together a series of yoga postures, customised for your needs, which can be practised before and/or after work. A lot of yoga teachers love working in this way; a way that is more aligned with how yoga was taught traditionally in India.

YOU WILL SEE MORE CLEARLY WHERE YOU HOLD STRESS IN YOUR BODY ...

This approach ensures that your practice of asanas will be tailored to your individual needs. Through working in an ongoing way with your teacher, you get to develop over time a personal practice appropriate for your body type, age and any underlying health conditions.

I include here a simple series of yoga stretches known as the Pawanmuktasana series, which I was taught through the Bihar School of Yoga. When done properly, these stretches can facilitate the free flow of prana around the body. This free flow of energy is gently encouraged by maintaining a conscious connection to your breath when doing the postures and by feeling into the part of the body being moved.

As your daily practice becomes more refined, you get to know your body better. You will see more clearly where you hold stress in your body and how that feels, and how it influences your thoughts and mood throughout the day. You will also be more able to recognise when physical, emotional and mental tension is starting to build up in your body and will know how to release that tension using these simple techniques.

Pawanmuktasana series of yoga postures

This is a series of gentle yoga postures designed to release wind energy (Vata dosha) held in the joints, and has a very balancing effect on the nervous system. This series is extremely useful in helping to prevent arthritis and joint stiffness. When doing these postures it is best to breathe through the nose in a relaxed yet focused way.

First, take a few moments to connect with your body, the earth beneath you and your breath. Set an intention for how you would like to approach your yoga practice. For example, if you are feeling speedy, your intention might be to do the practice slowly; if you are feeling lethargic and heavy your intention might be to do the practice vigorously; if you are feeling angry your intention might be to do the practice calmly. After each posture take a few moments to be aware of the effects of the practice on your body, mood and mind.

Wrist rotation With an outstretched right arm, rotate your wrist joint in a clockwise motion 10 times. Then rotate your wrist ten times in an anti-clockwise direction. Repeat the same movement with your left hand. On completion of the postures, allow your arms to rest beside your body.

Shoulder rotation With fingers touching the shoulders and elbows bent, make a circular movement from the shoulder joint, ten times clockwise, ten times anti-clockwise.

Pelvic rotation With your hands on your hips, rotate your pelvis in large circles. Do this ten times clockwise and ten times anti-clockwise.

Ankle rotation Standing on your left leg, raise your right leg, bent at the knee and draw circles with your right foot. Rotate the right foot clockwise ten times from the ankle joint. Then rotate the right foot anti-clockwise ten times. Repeat the procedure for the left foot.

Neck rotation Take a deep breath in and on the out-breath allow your head to gently drop down so that your chin almost touches your chest. Breathing in a relaxed way, slowly move your chin in a clockwise direction so that your chin draws a small circle. If you feel some tightness in the neck as you move around the clock, stop for a few moments and gently breathe into the tension in your neck, allowing it to soften and relax as you slowly breathe out. Then continue to move around the circle. Once you have finished two cycles in the clockwise direction, do two cycles in the anti-clockwise direction.

To finish, stand quietly for a few minutes, being aware of your whole body and feeling the effects of the practice on your body, mood and mind. This series of yoga postures is an excellent preparation for the practice of meditation.

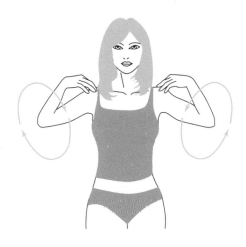

Adjusting your practice of asanas for your Ayurvedic body type

Vata-dominant body types generally do best with a calm, slow and gentle approach to their practice of asanas. Postures that work on the pelvis and colon, and which encourage elimination, are recommended. When undertaking their asana practice, it is important for them not to overexert themselves and to watch out for a feeling of depletion. There should be adequate rest and relaxation throughout their practice. Afterwards they should feel calm, warm and stable.

Pitta-dominant body types generally do best with a cooling, relaxed and expansive approach to their practice of asanas. Postures that work on the mid-abdomen, including the liver, are recommended. When undertaking their asana practice it is important for them not to force the posture and to watch out for overheating. They should adopt an attitude of relaxed enjoyment towards their practice and make sure they have plenty of time to sit quietly between stronger poses. Afterwards they should feel cool, calm and content.

Kapha-dominant body types generally do best with a stimulating, vigorous and creative approach to their practice of asanas. Postures that work on the chest and open up the heart and lungs are recommended. When undertaking their asana practice it is important for them not to take shortcuts and to watch out for avoidance of their practice and laziness. They need to keep their practice creative, and regularly bring in new poses and ways of doing them. Afterwards they should feel invigorated, warm and light.

Using your breath to stablilise your mind

In yoga, the breath is seen as the link between the mind and the body. When we are anxious and restless, our breath is erratic and shallow. When we are calm and relaxed, our breath is slower, deeper and more even. Through becoming more conscious of our breathing, we can influence the quality of our minds, making them clearer and quieter.

I became acutely aware of this principle many years ago on a day when my car registration and insurance was due. I had set aside several hours to go through the process of getting new tyres for my car and visiting the car insurance company and motor registry. As it turned out, that evening I was giving a three-hour talk on the anatomy and physiology of respiration, along with teaching some breathing exercises to a group of body-oriented psychotherapists in training.

I decided, as an experiment, to give my utmost attention to my breath during the whole time I was walking around the motor registry and interacting with various people. Whenever I possibly could I would direct my attention to my breath, not changing it in any way but simply being aware of it.

The results of this process were profound. Instead of approaching the day with a somewhat impatient agenda aimed at getting my car registered as quickly as possible, I found that I was much more relaxed as I moved around. I noticed with interest the architecture of the motor registry office, and also that I was much more available to the people I was dealing with. The quality of my interactions was innately satisfying, I was more in touch with my sense of humour and I found I actually enjoyed the time I spent re-registering my car rather than seeing it as a boring chore. At every step along the way, I was at the very centre of the unfolding process. There was no sense of time being wasted, rather a feeling that what I was doing was as good as anything else that I could be doing.

Training yourself to become more connected to your breath is an important aspect of yoga. It is known as pranayama, which means breath control. It is a simple and readily accessible way for us to be more present to the here and now, and to enjoy the benefits of a different way of being.

> TRAINING YOURSELF TO BECOME MORE CONNECTED TO YOUR BREATH IS AN IMPORTANT ASPECT OF YOGA.

Pranayama exercises work to purify the channels of energy in the pranic body, known as the pranamayakosha. They make us feel more energetic and, at the same time, more relaxed. This may at first seem like a contradiction, but when we are in a state of mind–body harmony or balance, both are present. We feel we have plenty of energy in reserve and there is also tremendous mental equipoise. During our practice of yogic breathing exercises we are consciously focusing our attention on our breath, diverting it away from the content of our thoughts, which is where our attention is focused most of the time.

You may be considering the state of your bank account, thinking about what you are going to have for dinner tonight or what your partner said to you this morning at breakfast. In pranayama, rather than getting caught up in these thoughts, you make the sensational awareness of your breath your primary concern. When thoughts such as these do wander into your conscious awareness, you gently but firmly return to your breath.

The regular practice of yogic breathing exercises helps to increase energy levels, enhances mental clarity and emotional stability, and supports the functioning of the nervous system. By dedicating a few minutes of your day to focussing on your breath, and not on the content of your consciousness, you will find that without any conscious effort on your part, you will be more aware of the quality of your breath throughout the day. You might notice, for example, when you have pulled up at the traffic lights that your shoulders are up around your ears and that you are holding your breath. With this newfound awareness, you can then choose to consciously breathe in and then breathe out slowly, allowing your shoulders to drop down to a more relaxed position. When you eventually get home, you will be in better shape both mentally and physically.

When practising pranayama, try to make sure that your head, neck and spine are aligned and your body relaxed. It is important to avoid straining as this can create headaches and neck strain. Generally it is best to practise a few hours after a meal and with an empty stomach and bladder. It is also important to practise in a well-ventilated room.

I include below two pranayama practices that are safe, easy to learn and appropriate for all body types. Pranayama practices work on a number of different levels, balancing our minds, our emotions and our physical bodies.

Conscious breathing exercise

Find a quiet place in your home where you are unlikely to be disturbed over the next fifteen minutes. This exercise can be done in a chair or sitting cross-legged on the floor.

Allow yourself to settle into a relaxed breathing pattern. Imagine that a rubber band is going from the top of your head towards the ceiling, gently elongating your spine. Bring your awareness to the act of breathing, specifically to the sensations in your nose and upper airways as you breathe in and out.

Allow your body to soften and relax. Feel the movement of the air through your nose and upper airways into your lungs. Feel the gentle rise and fall of your lungs with each breath in and out. Notice how that feels. Notice the quality of your breath. Is it regular or irregular, shallow or deep?

If your mind wanders off to other thoughts, gently bring it back to the sensations felt as you breathe in and out. Continue the practice for around five minutes and then just sit quietly, letting go of the focus on your breath and allowing it to roam freely.

Notice the effect of the practice on the quality of your thoughts, your mood and your physical body. Have they changed since the beginning of the practice?

Alternate nostril breathing

Sit comfortably in a chair with your feet firmly planted on the ground or cross-legged on the floor with your buttocks supported by a pillow. With a straight back, consciously relax your body. Hold the fingers of your right hand in front of your face. Rest the index and middle fingers on a spot midway between and slightly above your eyebrows. Close your eyes.

Close the right nostril with the thumb and breathe in through the left nostril with a normal level of inhalation. Then close the left nostril with the ring finger and breathe out through the right nostril. Then breathe in through the right nostril. Once your inhalation is complete, close it with the thumb and breathe out through the left nostril. This is one round.

Do five rounds in this way and then lower your hand and rest, quietly observing your breath. After a few minutes, do another five rounds and rest again. Once you have completed three rounds of five, sit quietly or lie down and observe your breathing in a passive way.

This practice is excellent for balancing the left and right hemispheres of the brain and has a sooting effect on the nervous system. It is an excellent preparation for meditation and is very useful if you suffer from insomnia.

Different types of pranayama practices

There are many kinds of pranayama practices, each one having different effects on the body–mind. Some types of pranayama, such as Ujjay pranayama, also known as the baby's snore breath, can easily be incorporated into your practice of yoga postures, whereas others are usually done sitting down after, or sometimes before, your practice of yoga postures. It is also possible to adjust your practice of pranayama so that it is in line with your Ayurvedic body type.

Alternate nostril breathing, as described, is good for all doshic types, though it is particularly recommended for Vata-dominant body types.

There are also yogic breathing exercises that involve inhaling through the mouth with a curled tongue or with the teeth clenched, which have a cooling effect on the body–mind. These are recommended for Pitta-dominant body types, especially during summer.

Some pranayama practices, such as the bellows breath, are more vigorous and involve rapid inhalation and exhalation of the lungs using the muscles of the diaphragm. This is a heating and stimulating practice that encourages purification of the lungs, it is particularly good for Kapha-dominant individuals.

As pranayama practices have a strong effect on the physiology of the body and mind, they need to be taught by a well-qualified teacher. Many yoga teachers are not overly experienced in pranayama, so make sure that your teacher has a long and well-established personal practice of pranayama, as well as plenty of experience in teaching it.

Suffice to say, yogic breathing exercises are a powerful complement to your practice of yoga postures and help to stabilise the mind prior to the practice of meditation. We will explore this idea in some detail in Chapter 7.

 Honouring the body – my yoga practice

Tracey is one of my previous students, a barrister by profession, who describes how the regular practice of yoga has impacted on her everyday life.

A yoga practice creates both time and space, because to hold a pose and really breathe when something is troubling you takes singular and present commitment.

Despite an understanding of this and years of practice, I often feel overwhelmed at the notion of putting aside the problem or focus of the day to practise. Yet once I start there is an uncanny quality in yoga that stands apart from the rest of my day while somehow still being able to relate to it. Each pose will always follow the last. I only have to do one pose at a time. To wonder what will come after 'reverse triangle' will mean I cannot give the pose the attention it deserves. To replay a frustrating meeting at work with a client or to make a mental grocery shopping list will almost certainly tip me off balance. To reach too hard for a pose will result in just that – reaching too hard. I know this but seem to need to be constantly reminded.

While on the mat during an asana, a thought might arise – if I can simply hold this pose for a fraction longer, I can handle that difficult situation tomorrow. Or, if I can surrender to a simple restorative posture it might be more challenging than a rigorous physical sequence.

My experience of yoga does not translate to some extraordinary transcendence into the divine. Yoga is not so earnest. It does not require hours of asanas and full lotus poses. It is not mere tranquillity. It is an evolving practice through which I have space to consider the quality of my awareness and perhaps, without realising, to create a spiritual dimension in the everyday.

The lost art of oil self-massage

Regular massaging of your body, known as abhyanga in Ayurveda, is another way of honouring your body and developing a more sensitive relationship with it. This helps foster a deeper connection with your body and benefits your health in a number of ways. Abhyanga encourages the circulation of blood and lymph around the body, improves dryness of the skin and makes the skin more lustrous, promotes strength and suppleness in the body and improves the quality of your sleep. It is a practice that can easily be incorporated into your daily routine, and it has a rejuvenating effect on both the mind and body.

While abhyanga is an important part of preventive medicine in Ayurveda and relevant to people of all ages, Ayurvedic texts also recommend oil self-massage for people whose health is too delicate to allow them to undertake physical exercise. It is therefore particularly relevant to the elderly, and I believe it has an important role to play in the field of aged care.

Depending on the dryness of your skin, you can use anywhere from two tablespoons to a quarter of a cup of oil. The choice of oil will depend on your body type and the season. In colder weather cold-pressed sesame oil is generally suitable for most people; in summer a cooling oil such as sunflower or coconut is more appropriate. For people with very oily skin, a light oil such as safflower oil or even a dry massage is recommended. For optimal results, the oil should be warmed prior to application. Placing the oil in a metal or porcelain cup and letting it sit in a bowl of hot water is a simple way to do this.

Abhyanga can be performed in the shower recess or sitting on a stool in the bathroom, depending on the amount of time you choose to spend doing it. A quick routine would involve getting into the shower, and letting the warm water cleanse your body and open up the pores of your skin. You can then give yourself a three-minute oil massage while standing up, before stepping back under the shower and washing off any residual oil from your skin. You can then towel dry and get dressed.

A longer routine might involve oiling up in a more leisurely way over ten or fifteen minutes while sitting on a stool or the side of the bath. It is important that you are warm at this time, so having a heater in the bathroom helps, especially in winter. Once you are oiled up, you can then put on some old clothes and walk around your home allowing the oil to absorb into the skin for the next few hours.

At the end of this time, depending on how much oil is left on your skin, you can have a quick shower and put on your usual clothes.

One student of mine, recognising that her skin and body were dry and had been for many years, decided to take up a daily practice of oil massage. She has a Vata-dominated body type, which is prone to dryness, so she chose to use sesame oil for the abhyanga. She diligently massaged a quarter of a cup of the oil into her body twice a day. It was not until the tenth day of this regime that she felt that her body was adequately oleated both internally and externally, given the previous state of the tissues of her body.

Technique for abhyanga

Start with your head, placing a small amount of oil on the flat of your hand and massaging the oil into the crown of your head. You can then massage the rest of your head using small circular movements with your fingers and palms. Alternatively, if you don't want to use so much oil, apply a few drops to your fingertips and massage your scalp as if shampooing your hair.

You can then move downwards applying the oil to your face, the front and back of the neck and the shoulders and arms. When massaging the upper and

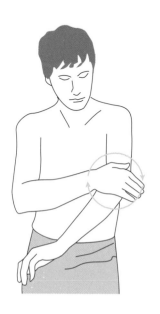

lower limbs it is best to use circular movements over the joints and a back and forth movement over the long bones. Next, apply the oil to the front of the chest and the parts of your back that you can reach. When massaging the abdomen, use a gentle circular motion following the large bowel from right to left across the abdomen. The back, spine and legs are then massaged and finally the soles of the feet.

The head and the soles of the feet have a dense concentration of marma, or vital points, which, when stimulated, have a reflex effect on the internal organs and other parts of your body. It is therefore particularly worthwhile spending extra time massaging the scalp and feet.

Tim's story: the joy of oil

I asked my colleague Tim Mitchell, with whom I taught Ayurvedic cooking classes, to share his passion for abhyanga. He gives a heartfelt account of the delights for body, mind and spirit from self-oil massage.

The eastern sky is lightening above the horizon as I arrive at the beach. On the southern edge a saltwater pool nestles at base of the sandstone cliffs. Already a couple of slow steady swimmers are in the water, and outside the pool in the ocean a surfer catches his first wave. The air is chilly and being winter, the water will prove to be even more so.

I roll out my yoga mat and unzip my Ayurvedic beach bag – a thermos of ginger tea, a mug and a bottle of oil (sesame or almond, or coconut in summer). After pouring a cup of tea I put the oil bottle in the cup to warm the oil and undress to my bathers. With the oil now warm, and after some sips of ginger tea, I apply the oil all over my body and then come back and rub my whole body in sequence with the simple Ayurvedic strokes: long, light strokes on the long bones and circles over the joints, from the feet and hands in towards the heart.

Against the cool winter air the warm oil is soothing. Some of it soaks in. The sun's healing rays glisten on oily skin as I perform a salute to the sun, a sequence of yoga postures, for a few minutes. Already the oil protects me from the sharpness of the air and, while many in the pool wear wetsuits, I wear just a swim cap as again the oil lessens the shock of the cold water. After ten or fifteen minutes of laps I am thankful for the warm showers in the public amenities (the local mayor swims here every morning!) and with minimal soap I wash the remaining oil from my skin and go happily into my day.

If you do this you will catch far fewer colds and flu than your workmates. Your skin will not need expensive moisturisers. You will be protected from hostile environments, like air-conditioning. It strengthens all the tissues of the body and enhances removal of toxins and wastes. It promotes peaceful sleep and good vision, too. It is a time-honoured practice in India to encourage longevity. It reduces anxiety and the effect of stress.

It took me a long time to incorporate oil self-massage into my daily routine, after a decade of knowing about it through my love and study of Ayurveda. Along with yoga and meditation it is now a pillar of my daily investment in my health. And apart from all of the above, it feels great to care for yourself like this. I urge you to try it for just one week, maybe for just four days of the week, and see how you feel at the end. Experience is the greatest teacher.

Counterbalancing the effects of technology on the body

From the perspective of Ayurveda, time spent on computers, tablets, mobile phones and computer games increases and can potentially aggravate Vata dosha. Vata dosha controls the nervous system and too much screen time is inherently stimulating to the nervous system. This needs to be balanced in practical ways.

The Ayurvedic principle of moderation in all things applies when it comes to computer use, though this is a challenging thing to practise in the current age. It is, however, possible to prevent Vata dosha going out of balance in two main ways.

1. Implementing health-giving strategies for how you use technology which prevent the build-up of Vata dosha in the body in the first place. Setting up a health-promoting workspace is an important starting point. A room that is well lit with the ability to look past your screen and out of a window is essential. A comfortable, ergonomically designed chair that supports a good posture is also important.

Health tip

A hot shower and oil self-massage is a great way to balance Vata dosha after working on the computer.

Taking regular breaks every 20 minutes from your work will reduce the build-up of muscle tension in the body and eyestrain. During the breaks you might choose to walk around your office or home, do a few gentle stretches, interact with a work colleague, drink a glass of warm water or cup of herbal tea or go to the toilet. If your workplace is air-conditioned it is important to stay well hydrated. Warm water or herbal tea helps in this regard and also balances Vata dosha, which is cold in nature. When you sit still and work on a computer, the body cools down and the circulation becomes sluggish. Gentle stretching and movement stimulates the flow of prana around the body and helps you feel less fatigued.

2. After spending time on the computer, you can incorporate specific measures to antidote increases in Vata dosha. A warm to hot shower incorporating a quick oil massage, as described earlier in this chapter, is a great combination. Other Vata-pacifying activities include gentle yoga stretches such as the Pawanmuktasana series, going for a walk around the block, gardening, walking barefoot on grass,

going for a swim and drinking a cup of warm soup. Contact with nature is inherently balancing to Vata dosha and helps to ground the energy of the body.

Ayurveda recommends limiting your computer use after dark, but if you do need to work at night it is best to stop two hours before going to bed. This will help you to sleep more soundly and reduces the risk of insomnia. If, for some reason, you have had to spend a lot of time on the computer over an extended period, consider giving your body a present in the form of a massage, a reflexology treatment, a day at the beach or a weekend bushwalk. These activities all help to pacify Vata dosha and ground the energy of your body-mind.

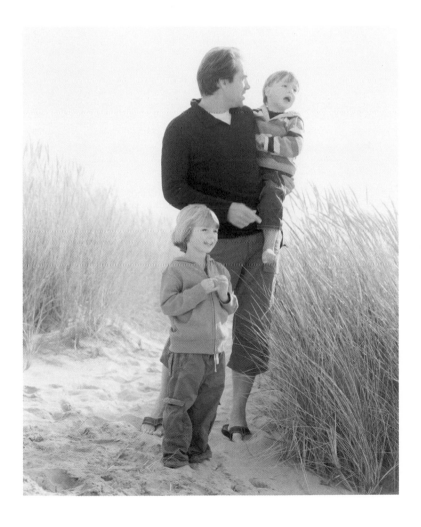

chapter 6

Cultivating a quiet mind

Happiness is inherent in man and not due to external causes. One must realise his Self in order to open the store of unalloyed happiness.

Ramana Maharshi

Most of us have visited places that have a profoundly quietening effect on the mind. Places where the atmosphere is so refined that even the most active or disturbed mind is quickly soothed and feels at peace. Many years ago, while travelling with a couple of friends in India, I had my own experience of this at the ancient Buddhist caves at Ajanta in Maharashtra state.

The caves are located on the sides of a narrow gorge and have been cut out from the rock cliff face. They date back to the second century BCE and were home to Buddhist monks, scholars, sculptors and painters over several centuries. Uninhabited for centuries, the caves had become covered by jungle and were only rediscovered in 1819 by an English officer on a tiger hunting expedition.

Our visit to Ajanta coincided with the arrival of a busload of young Tibetan monks who, under the careful supervision of a venerable old lama, were on a pilgrimage to the caves. They invited us to join them, which we did, and watched in awe as they performed full-length prostrations at the feet of the enormous, elaborately carved Buddhas and Bodhisattvas on the dusty floors of the caves. Their enthusiastic and heartfelt offerings left an indelible impression on our Western eyes, less accustomed to such overt acts of religious devotion.

Some of the caves were actually monasteries, complete with a central hall surrounded by cells where the monks lived and meditated. The larger caves extended 50 metres into the hillside, and offered a welcome relief from the heat outside. As the young monks had moved onto the next cave, I decided to sit for a few minutes in one of the cells, on the level surface provided by a bed cut from rock.

Despite the arduous trip getting to the caves, as soon as I closed my eyes, I could feel the stillness of the hill envelope me. It was as if my mind had been instantly deactivated and the usual train of incessant thoughts had somehow disappeared. Transported to another realm, quite impossible to describe, it was difficult to find the will to get up and rejoin the rest of the group. Later that day, I was left to imagine the lives of the monks who had lived and meditated in these caves for so many centuries, firm in the conviction that their refined presence lives on in these subterranean caverns.

So how can we cultivate a quiet mind in an increasingly fast-paced and frenetic world? A world driven by technological advances and where our minds are exposed to hitherto unimagined levels of stimulation. In this chapter I would like to focus on how you can connect with your innate stillness and inner calm by developing a daily practice of meditation.

> SO HOW CAN WE CULTIVATE A QUIET MIND IN AN INCREASINGLY FAST-PACED AND FRENETIC WORLD?

In the traditional education of a yoga and meditation teacher in India, your apprenticeship initially entails duties such as cleaning the yoga hall and helping with the day-to-day running of the yoga school. You would also undergo several years of training in yoga postures (asanas), closely supervised by your teacher. After several years of asana training, you would be introduced to yogic breathing exercises known as pranayama. Then when you had completed a few years of combining yoga postures and breathing exercises in a daily morning practice, and when your teacher felt you were ready, you would be introduced to the practice of meditation. The training was reliant on a close relationship between teacher and student, and was customised for the individual needs of the apprentice.

I mention this to give some idea of the context in which meditation was taught and practised. In simple terms, there was a strong emphasis on preparing the body–mind prior to the practice of meditation. The student's body was enlivened through the practice of yoga postures and he or she developed the capacity to sit comfortably and steadily for long periods of time. This was deemed a necessary requirement for deeper meditation practices. Yogic breathing exercises helped to purify the body–mind and had a stabilising effect on the student's thought processes. They also functioned to develop a greater awareness of the link between the quality of the student's breath and the quality of their mind.

In modern times, however, meditation has become a commodity for sale and is often taught with little or no attention to these principles. Students can do a weekend intensive, be given their mantra or a particular practice and away they go. Sometimes no provision is made to enable the student to have an ongoing relationship with their teacher. Little wonder then that they are unable to reap the benefits of meditation and it falls into the too-hard basket or simply gets lost in that person's life.

In my medical practice, as part of an holistic assessment, I often ask patients about their experience with meditation. Over the years, many have said that they know meditation would be good for them, but they have been unable to establish a regular practice in their lives, despite having done several short courses. Others say that they find it difficult to stop the incessant stream of thoughts even while meditating. One woman complained that she was even more neurotically aware of her worries and concerns after 20 minutes of meditation than she was before starting her practice. Certainly, it is my experience that many people are not experiencing the full benefits of the practice of meditation and hence have either lost interest in it or feel that they are somehow a lost cause and meditation is not for them.

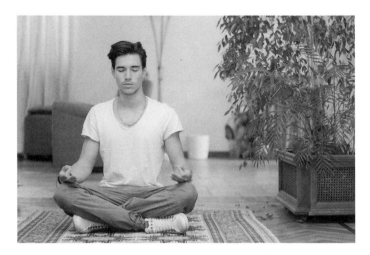

Defining meditation

In meditation you train the mind by focusing your attention on something. This can be anything from a bodily sensation, a sacred sound or mantra, your breath, a candle flame or a mental creation. Over the millennia lots of different objects have been used to help focus the mind in different spiritual and healing traditions. In India, the nature of the mind is understood to be restless activity. The mind is often referred to as the 'monkey mind', because of its tendency to refuse to do what is asked of it, and seemingly it has its own innate agenda.

In meditation this natural tendency of the mind is accepted rather than fought against, as fighting to control the mind with your will only adds fuel to the mind. The mind is seen as a bundle of thoughts and your thought to control it simply fattens up the mind, much like throwing sticks on to a fire.

When you sit to practise meditation, after some time your mind will naturally wander from the nominated focus to some other thought. At this point you gently but firmly bring your attention back to the agreed focus. When the mind again wanders, you again bring it back to the focus.

Through this ebb and flow, the practice of meditation acts as a vehicle taking us from the busy superficial levels of the mind down to the quieter, deeper levels of the mind.

Many years ago, I taught meditation to a middle-aged man with no previous experience in meditation. I guided him through an awareness meditation, focussing on sensations around his body and his breath. I had the sense that he had quite a deep experience during the 25 minutes of the guided meditation. Afterwards I asked him about his experience and all he could say was, 'I have just been someplace else.' Certainly he looked very relaxed and at peace from the practice, but was unable to say anything more about his experience. Not everyone has such a calming first experience of meditation – a lot of people need to work at it for many years before it starts to reveal its magic.

Since the 1970s there has been a significant amount of scientific research into meditation, which has demonstrated that there are measurable physiological changes in the body and mind that are associated with the meditative state. Dr Herbert Benson, a professor of behavioural medicine at Harvard University, did a lot of the pioneering research into meditation in the 1970s and coined the term 'The Relaxation Response' to describe the meditative state. He and other researchers were able to demonstrate slowing down of the heart and respiratory rates, a reduction in blood pressure, changes in brain wave activity when measured by an electroencephalogram, and a shift in activity from the left to the right hemisphere of the brain during meditation.

In the last decade there has also emerged a growing body of research using the latest neural imaging technologies into the neurobiology of meditation. This is demonstrating that there are measurable changes in brain functioning and structure in experienced meditators.

Finding the right meditation for you

Learning to meditate is an oral tradition. It is learnt in the context of a student–teacher relationship that is fundamental in helping the student progress and experience the full benefits of their practice. Thus it is important to find a teacher who you have a good feeling about, who seems to be walking their talk and who inspires you in some way. As mentioned, if the teacher is interested in having an ongoing association with you as a student, this helps enormously.

The meditation practice that really appeals to you and engages you is undoubtedly the practice to pursue. This is where your intuition can be a wonderful guide. Making a commitment to maintain your practice for a reasonable length of time will help you know, further down the track, whether this is the practice for you.

There are many different types of meditation practices including those focused on mantras or sacred sounds, body awareness, mental visualisations, chanting and candle gazing to name only a few. Most involve sitting or kneeling, while some can be done lying down such as yoga nidra, in which your awareness is systematically moved around your body. Exposing yourself to a few different traditions can be helpful in finding what feels right for you.

At a practical level, it is also important to make some kind of assessment of whether the suggested practice can be reasonably integrated into your daily routine. If the tradition strongly recommends that you sit for an hour a day, it may not be something that is doable in the context of where you are at in your life. Rather than commit to something that is likely to fail, it is better to look around for a meditation practice that can more easily be incorporated into your current lifestyle.

Establishing a personal practice of meditation

Finding an appropriate place in your home to practice meditation will help support your personal practice. Many people choose an area in their bedroom as it tends to be more quiet and private; some may devote a room in the house expressly for the purpose of meditation and spiritual practice. As you continue to meditate there you will find that a subtle change in the vibrational quality of that part of the room will be more and more apparent. Through your ongoing practice of meditation an energetic field is created that has a transformative effect on the body–mind. As with the meditation chambers used by the monks at Ajanta, the quality of the field is such that it helps you go to a deeper place in your meditation.

In terms of preparing yourself for meditation, I have spoken of the benefits of yoga postures and yogic breathing exercises – practices that encourage the flow of prana in the body. Exercise that encourages you to connect with your body and breath, such as walking and swimming, is also very useful. These activities will help get you out of your head and serve to revitalise your body, and in this way support you in having a satisfying experience of meditation. A practice of meditation that you naturally want to experience each day and for which you will happily set aside some time.

Most meditation practices are done sitting or kneeling, though for some people a lying down practice is most appropriate. In the awareness meditation I teach, you lie down on your back and move your awareness from head to toe, focusing your mind on sensations in the body. As a medical doctor I find this style of meditation is particularly helpful with patients who are suffering from some kind of physical illness, as it encourages rest and rejuvenation. It also allows the nervous system and digestive tract to relax deeply. Importantly, it can help people learn how to rest, a largely forgotten concept in the Western world where so many people are running on nervous energy and caffeine and rarely allow themselves to stop.

The length of time of your meditation practice is also worth considering. Some traditional practices encourage an hour of meditation at each sitting, but many people will simply not be able to find a block of time this long in their daily routine, particularly when they are caring for young children. Many of the parents I see in my consultations find mini-meditations extremely useful. Just to stop for a few minutes, perhaps lie down on their bed, connect with their body and any tension held in it and to breathe more consciously can be a great circuit breaker of stress. After only a few minutes, they emerge a little more centred, less overwhelmed and with a greater sense of control in their lives.

Some people feel that unless they can sit for the prescribed 20 minutes, they may as well not bother with their meditation practice. However, a flexible approach that takes into account the amount of time available to you on a given day will help to ensure that meditation happens every day in some form or another. In this sense, mini-meditations should not be underestimated in their value.

An example of a mini-meditation

Connect with yourself by sitting quietly with your feet on the ground and eyes closed. Consciously let go of wherever you have come from – physically, emotionally and mentally. Feel your body from the top of the head to the tips of the toes, noticing any areas of discomfort or pleasure. Feel your connection with the ground beneath you, the solidness of Mother Earth. Notice the quality of your breath. Is it regular or irregular, shallow or deep? Become aware of your senses of hearing, taste, touch and smell. Ask yourself the simple question, 'How am I feeling?' And wait for the answer that comes, without having to think about it. Slowly come back into the room and into relationship with other people and the outside world. Allow your eyes to open when you feel ready. Remember to be gentle with yourself, always gentle.

Some tips to help you into a satisfying practice of meditation

- Look at your daily routine and work out the best time or times in your day to meditate, and try to meditate at around the same time each day initially.
- Avoid meditating on a full stomach, which is likely to promote drowsiness
- Find a quiet place in your house where you are unlikely to be disturbed. In order to minimise potential disturbance, you may want to turn your mobile phone off, put the telephone answering machine on or put a 'Do not disturb sign' on your bedroom door.

- Make sure you feel comfortable. Removing jewellery, watches and belts helps in this process. A warm shawl to cover yourself is useful especially in winter.
- You might like to start your meditation practice with a ritual of some kind such as lighting a candle or incense, or placing a flower on an altar.
- Centre yourself prior to meditation by taking three slow, deep breaths in and out through the nose.
- Try to let go of any expectations prior to starting your meditation practice; this will help in allowing you to be more open to whatever experience comes.
- The basic attitude in meditation is 'the journey is the goal'.
- Whatever happens always remember to be gentle with yourself.
- Allow five to ten minutes at the end of your meditation practice to slowly come back into the room before going on to the next part of your day.

Mindfulness

Mindfulness is a Buddhist practice in which you consciously choose to bring your awareness to the present moment rather than getting involved in the content of your thoughts. In recent times, it has become popular in the West through the work of Dr Jon Kabat-Zinn and is being used therapeutically to help people with pain, anxiety, depression and stress. The practice is based around paying complete attention to each thought, feeling and sensation that is arising in the field of your awareness. Whatever arises is acknowledged and accepted just as it is. The regular practice of mindfulness allows your mind to soften and opens you to the unfolding moment – whatever it may bring.

When learning the practice, it is useful to set aside periods of time where you sit quietly and are mindful in this way. The beauty of this practice is that it can be extended into your everyday life, as an ongoing state of mind. When practised over time, it helps you recognise habitual patterns of thinking and allows for the possibility of new ways of responding to situations and events in your life. I include below an introductory exercise in mindfulness.

Mindfulness exercise

Sit quietly in a comfortable chair with your feet firmly planted on the ground. Feel your connection with the earth.

Bring your attention to your physical body. Be aware of sensations on your skin, in your muscles and within your body. Notice where you feel warmth or coolness, tightness or softness, lightness or heaviness, etc. Observe without judging or commenting on your experience.

Next bring your attention to your breath, focusing on the subtle sensations as air passes in and out of your nostrils and upper airways. Enjoy the simple act of breathing, without any restriction or strain.

Be aware of the sounds around you. Notice that whatever you hear comes to your ears without any effort on your part. Allow sounds to wash over you in their own random way.

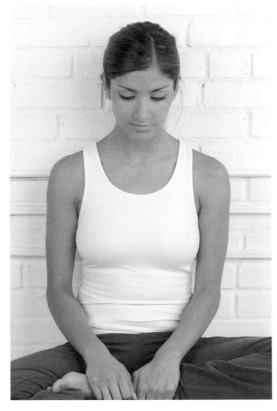

Then direct your attention to thoughts that are arising. Some may have strong emotions associated with them, some not. See them as passing phenomena and allow them to come and go, much like clouds passing across the sky. They come and they go. When your mind wanders from the present moment, gently bring it back to your breath.

Continue to sit in this way for ten to fifteen minutes, being with yourself and your unfolding experience. Remember to be gentle with yourself, always gentle.

Afterwards sit quietly with yourself or lie down, noticing the effects of the practice on the quality of your thoughts, your mood and your physical body.

Supporting your practice of meditation

Listening to meditation CDs, podcasts and apps on your smart phone can be extremely helpful in supporting a personal practice of meditation. They can also be a useful stepping stone for beginners wanting to acquaint themselves with a meditation practice. Meditation CDs also have the advantage of allowing you to receive the guided practice, which is particularly useful when you are tired from a long day at work or parenting at home. Nothing is required of you other than to listen and follow the words of the teacher as best you can. This kind of practice can be very restorative and is particularly appropriate when there is depletion or fatigue.

Attending group meditation evenings and meditation retreats, particularly in the tradition you have been taught in, can help sustain your personal practice. Many people find that being part of group meditation allows their experience of meditation to go deeper. It also provides an opportunity to connect with like-minded people and to receive guidance from your teacher about your practice and address any concerns you may have about your experiences.

 My practice of meditation

Judy, a yoga and meditation teacher, shares her daily practice of meditation; one she has fine-tuned over many years that connects her to her essential nature.

Gaining the discipline to stay focused during meditation takes practice. I have learnt to observe when I become distracted by thoughts, feelings or bodily distractions and return my awareness back to the point of focus (again and again). Being gentle and patient with myself helps. Whenever I experience 'resistance' to commence meditating or during meditation, I have learnt to form a relationship with the resistance and become curious to sit with it, to face the resistance rather than avoid it. Usually, a limiting pattern will be exposed and the resistance dissolves. I actively cultivate an attitude of curiosity towards meditation so that my meditation practice does not become a chore. Dedicating my meditation practice to greater consciousness in the world also strengthens my commitment.

I have derived many personal benefits from my meditation practice. Physical tensions have dissolved, and I have developed a greater breath capacity. I'm able to discern between present moment feelings versus old emotional patterns, and reactivity and defensiveness that are the results of my mind's commentary. A greater awareness of my conditioning, being in touch with my needs, awareness of the inner critic, catching worrying about the future and being stuck in the past are all valuable insights that I have gained. When managing life's challenges, I have greater emotional resilience, mental clarity and a sense of connectedness to the greater forces of universal energy.

During meditation, I arrive at a place where I meet myself and then go beyond my ego and experience a deeper connection to my divine essence. Stillness is always below the thin surface of my thoughts. When I become quiet, I hear the voice of my soul. I open up to what I express as Oneness, Inspiration and Love.

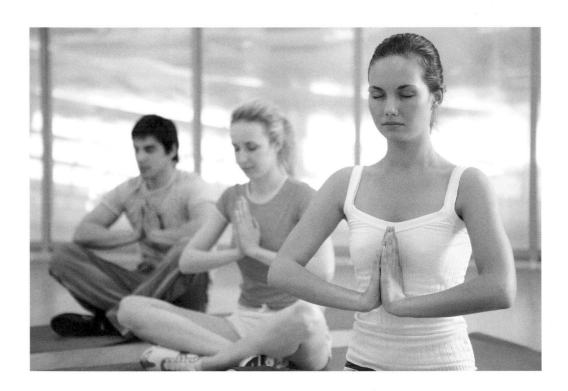

Chapter 7

Connecting with spirit

Your true nature is beyond description. It cannot be known with the mind, yet it exists. It is the source of everything.

Nisargadatta Maharaj

•

It was dusk on New Year's Eve and a group of 150 people, mostly families, were sitting around the makeshift stage watching a group of local Aboriginal dancers and musicians sharing traditional stories from their country. They were proud Bundgelung men clad in ochre and you could see how much the sharing of their stories meant to them. The place was Byron Bay and the setting some parkland just above the beach near the centre of town. In the failing light, you could just make out the grey slip of beach spreading east in a long arc to the promontory of Cape Byron. Above us, hundreds of rainbow lorikeets were screeching and carrying on in the huge Norfolk Island Pines creating a raucous background to the scene we were witnessing.

At the end of the performance, the head dancer came to the microphone and spoke to the assembled gathering. He thanked the crowd for being there and acknowledged the spirit of the land we were standing on. 'You can feel that spirit now,' he announced to the mostly non-Indigenous mums, dads and children sitting on the grass in front of him.

As he spoke these words, I felt the truth of what he was saying. I felt it through my whole body. An unmistakeable experience that is impossible to adequately describe, but once felt leaves a lasting impression. It was as if he was telling us, on a sunny day, that the sun is shining. It was so patently obvious and true that it hardly bears mentioning. I had the distinct impression that I was not the only person in the crowd that warm summer evening who was feeling the import of his words, and was, at least in that moment, aligned with spirit.

In this chapter I explore some of the ways of aligning with spirit that come to us from the ancient tradition of yoga. The word yoga comes from the root word 'yuj' in Sanskrit, which means to yoke or unite. In this sense, yoga is concerned with how to yoke yourself with the divine in your daily life, how to become one with the process of life itself.

The word yoga, in Western countries at least, is usually associated with the practice of yoga postures, though this is only a small part of yoga. In India, today, yoga is more likely to be understood as a process involving different forms of spiritual practice that leads to enlightenment. In India, there exists a large number of yogic paths, many of which have lineages that go back over thousands of years.

Your true nature

Yoga holds that your essential nature is peace; a quality of being that becomes self-evident when your mind is still and your emotions are calm. When your mind is very active and your mood is changeable, it is difficult to feel that inner peace and harmony. In this reactive state we get embroiled in the dramas of our lives and suffer as a result.

In order to counter this tendency, yoga recommends that you develop a daily sadhana or spiritual practice to help you reconnect with your true nature. Often this will involve a formal period of time during the day in which you devote yourself to spiritual practices you are drawn to. However, the aim of spiritual practice is to integrate its approaches into all aspects of your life, including your relationships at home, at work and at large.

What kind of spiritual practice you are drawn to and decide to take on is a highly individual affair. In many traditions of yoga the student is given specific spiritual practice by a teacher or guru. This usually involves a series of practices that are individually tailored for the needs of that student and which work with the body, mind and spirit. It is also true that for some people their spiritual practice is a much less structured affair that they refine for themselves over time.

In modern times when there are so many different schools of yoga on offer in the marketplace, it can be difficult to know where to start. I encourage people to sit down and articulate for themselves what they really want from their spiritual practice. Once you have clarity around this, it is important to stay open and expose yourself to different yogic and other spiritual traditions, whether they come from Christianity, Buddhism, Islam or Hinduism.

Which one feels right intuitively? Does it resonate with your core values and allow you to connect with the deepest part of yourself? Ultimately the tradition that speaks to your heart will be the right one for you, though this may well change over time, as you develop and grow as a human being.

In the following sections I give a brief overview of the four main paths described in yoga, what they look like and what kinds of people are likely to be attracted to them. The four paths are karma, bhakti, raja and jnana yoga and are designed to suit different human temperaments. The paths are certainly not mutually exclusive and in many ways complement each other.

You may find that one path has the strongest appeal for you or that all four paths resonate with you in some way. All types of combinations are possible and will be reflected in the spiritual practice you establish for yourself. It is important to say that there are many other paths of yoga, existing as vibrant traditions in India and around the world, though a more thorough examination of them is beyond the scope of this book. In the words of Mahatma Gandhi, 'Truth is one, paths are many.'

Karma yoga – the path of social service

Karma yoga tends to be attractive to people with an active disposition, people who see a practical problem and want to do something about it. Importantly, in karma yoga, work is undertaken in a spirit of non-attachment to the fruits of your actions. In other words, you give yourself entirely to the task at hand, making your best effort, but do so with the utter conviction that how it will turn out is ultimately not in your hands. The outcome is seen to be in God's hands, not yours.

Karma yoga encourages you to stay present to the process, rather than getting too involved in the end result. How things turn out is left to the divine and is essentially not your concern. The approach of Karma yoga can be brought into each and every action of your day. It involves bringing as much awareness and effort as you can muster to what you are doing and being attentive to the present moment. In this way, the details of each step along the way are being attended to mindfully. As the outcome is understood to be beyond your control, there is not the same pressure driving the work, which in itself allows for a gentler approach. Your actions become more graceful and the people you are working with benefit from your relaxed presence.

I am often inspired by people I know who have taken on voluntary work in the spirit of Karma yoga. Some serve food at a hostel for homeless men, others work with women in crisis at a women's refuge, and still others train women caught up in the sex industry in Cambodia to become yoga teachers and find alternative employment. It is obvious to me that for them, the voluntary work is its own reward.

Mahatma Gandhi was a great example of someone who practised karma yoga. He often said that his life was his message, a life that included his work in helping India get its independence from the British. At various stages in that struggle, it involved him speaking at public rallies, negotiating with other independence leaders, going to gaol and even undertaking hunger fasts. One of the verses on karma yoga in the Bhagavadgita, one of India's most sacred texts, was a favourite of his and a guiding principle in his life. It captures the essence of karma yoga.

> *To action alone hast thou a right and never to its fruits;*
> *Let not the fruits of action be thy motive;*
> *Neither let there be in thee any attachment to inaction.*

Bhagavadgita II, 47.

Bhakti yoga – the path of devotion

Bhakti yoga is by far the most popular path of yoga in India today and appeals to people with a strong felt sense of the divine in all aspects of life. For them it is quite natural to want to devote themselves to the worship and service of God.

In Hinduism the divine may be in the form of a specific deity such as Shiva or Krishna, or an enlightened spiritual teacher. In contemporary Bhakti yoga, the devotion may be to the form of the Beloved that most touches your heart.

In Bhakti yoga there is a very close and personal relationship with the Godhead and various forms of worship are prescribed. These may include devotional singing and the chanting of mantras, which encourage the heart to open. Spiritual practices such as these may be associated with altered states of consciousness, profound epiphanies and intense feelings of love for God. Other forms of worship include specific rituals and acts of service where the devotee puts their personal needs aside, surrendering them to God.

Through ongoing acts of personal surrender, the devotee seeks to become one with the object of their worship. He or she admits that they are lost without the help of their Beloved. In this spirit, all responsibility for your spiritual welfare is handed over to God. Whatever experiences befall you are seen as an expression of God's will and accepted in that light. An illness or car accident, as well as any successes in life are understood as coming from the divine and not cause for personal castigation or pride. The changing circumstances of your life are viewed as opportunities to open to a more loving connection with God.

This path requires a great deal of trust and is extremely uncomfortable for many people. It involves a conscious letting go of your sense of personal control and requires a high degree of vulnerability from the point of view of the individual. Necessarily it can open the way to abuses of power and the spiritual scene is littered with examples of gurus taking advantage of their devotees and their families. That said, it is generally accepted that the Indian psyche has a much greater capacity for Bhakti yoga, when compared with the Western mind where the need for individual autonomy is deeply entrenched.

Raja yoga – the path of the mystic

Raja yoga refers to a path of spiritual development with eight limbs, laid out in a yogic text known as the Yoga Sutra, written by the sage Patanjali in the second century CE. This path involves ethical and moral trainings as well as focusing on yoga postures (asanas), yogic breathing techniques (pranayama) and various kinds of concentration exercises culminating in meditation and deep connection with the divine.

The structure inherent in this path is very attractive to individuals with a natural sensitivity to their own internal experience, which is perhaps why it has been traditionally called the path of the mystic.

Initially there is a strong focus on yoga postures that develop the capacity to sit comfortably for long periods of time in order to facilitate meditation. The mind is then made steady through yogic breathing practices. Later the ability to develop a single point of mental concentration is cultivated. This in turn prepares the way for states of absorption where the meditator becomes one with the object of meditation: a place of bliss known as samadhi.

Many schools of yoga in the West draw from the traditions of Raja yoga, though often they will focus more on trainings involving the body and the breath. Each school will emphasise slightly different aspects of the tradition, depending on the lineage and inclinations of the teacher. Some of these schools may also bring in practices from the other paths of yoga.

Hatha yoga is generally held to be a preparatory path for Raja yoga. It aims to purify the body using various yogic practices, including asanas, pranayama exercises and salt water cleansing techniques.

Jnana yoga – the path of wisdom

Jnana yoga generally appeals to people who are psychologically minded with a natural capacity for introspection. It holds that our primary problem is a case of mistaken identity, essentially that we take ourselves to be what we are not. We identify ourselves with our bodies with all their accompanying conditioning rather than with our true nature, which is timeless and changeless. This tradition differentiates the self, which is bound by name, age, gender and social status from the Self, which is unbounded and limitless.

Having identified ourselves with our bodies, we take our false identity into the world and the drama of our life unfolds in its own unique way from that point. In Jnana yoga, you are encouraged to go to the source of your I-centred thoughts, rather than getting caught up with all the ups and downs of the person you have taken yourself to be. In this tradition, also known as Self-Enquiry, you are encouraged to ask, 'Who is feeling angry right now? Who is feeling frightened? Who is feeling proud?'

Instead of giving energy to the ego's needs, you actually undermine the ego, coming back to your essential spiritual nature. A place of effortless being where your sense of individuality has fallen away and only peace remains. Initially this type of enquiry is done during periods of formal practice though ultimately it can be practised throughout the day, regardless of what type of activity you are engaged in doing.

Jnana yoga often involves attending satsangs, where the teaching proceeds through question and answer sessions. The presence and words of the teacher helps the understanding to go deeper in the hearts and minds of the student. The student is then encouraged to go away and contemplate the teachings, both actively and passively, in the context of their lived experience.

The path of Jnana yoga may involve reading spiritual texts, both ancient and contemporary, from teachers in this tradition. Initially an intellectual understanding of the approach is required. Later, that understanding needs to be integrated into your being through practice. In India today and around the world, there exist many teachers of Jnana yoga with varying degrees of understanding and authenticity.

Ramana Maharshi, who lived at the base of the holy mountain of Arunachala in South India for most of his life, is generally acknowledged as the foremost teacher of Jnana yoga in the 20th century. He, more than any other, is responsible for popularising the enquiry, 'Who am I?' In his talks with spiritual seekers from all over the world he would encourage people to go back to the source of their thoughts and to reside there, remaining with the 'I' thought. In the words of Ramana Maharshi, 'If you hold this feeling of "I" long enough and strongly enough, the false "I" will vanish, leaving only the unbroken awareness of the real, immanent "I", consciousness itself.'

Nourishing your spiritual practice

Your spiritual practice, like any other part of your life, needs to be regularly nourished and enlivened. Here I discuss various ways that are traditionally advocated to support your spiritual practice.

Satsang, or 'keeping the company of the wise', is one of the main ways of supporting your spiritual life. In practice it has a number of different forms. It may involve a question and answer session with a spiritual adept, listening to a spiritual discourse or just simply sitting quietly in the presence of a realised being.

While studying Ayurveda in India, one of my senior lecturers mentioned to me that part of his spiritual practice involved visiting a young man acknowledged as a highly refined spiritual adept. Despite having a busy schedule at the university and a young family, he would find time on the weekends to visit the young sage. He and a small group of other spiritual aspirants would simply sit in silence in the same room as the young man for hours at a time.

This kind of satsang has long been a part of the spiritual traditions of India. The purity of the energy field around such beings creates the conditions for aspirants to have deeper experiences in meditation and profound insights into their own nature and life itself.

Yogic texts and tradition also speak of the need for spiritual community, known as sangha, to support spiritual life. In order to facilitate the process of physical, emotional and mental refinement, the presence of like-minded people in your day-to-day life is given a high priority. In traditional Indian society, the local temple would provide a strong focus for activities that nurture the spirit and offer opportunities to interact with people of spiritual inclination. In contemporary Western society, I see people finding spiritual community in a variety of settings such as personal development seminars, twelve-step programs, yoga schools, and religious groups such as Christian fellowships, Islamic study groups and Buddhist sanghas.

What I observe in true spiritual community is that people feel free to express themselves more authentically and without fear of judgement. You tend to be taken at face value by others and do not have to deal with family and cultural rules about how you should think and behave. The people in the community have a personal commitment to a vision that is greater than themselves; a vision that honours the individuality of each person in the group and is not invested in wanting you to conform to a predetermined set of expectations. Importantly, groups with these qualities help engender self-exploration and self-acceptance, a cornerstone of spiritual growth.

Over the last fifteen years I have coordinated a two-year program in Ayurvedic medicine for people studying to become Ayurvedic lifestyle consultants. During that time I have met thousands of students, some of whom have come to the college with significant personal problems. The problem may relate to difficulties with physical or mental health and/or relationship breakdown.

Sometimes I will have a student of this kind early in their course of studies and after teaching them for a few months they go on to study other courses in the college of natural therapies. Not infrequently I have had the experience of bumping into them at the college cafeteria several years later, and am barely able to recognise them, such is the change in their posture and demeanour. They often appear to be lighter and happier, and it is obvious that a profound transformation has taken place in their lives. There is also a real sense that this transformation was a product of the positive interactions they were having with their teachers and fellow students. They were now part of a community that supported their growth and development as human beings, which had become an integral part of their daily life.

Pilgrimage

Pilgrimage to holy places, known as 'yatra' in Sanskrit, is also traditionally recommended as a way of supporting spiritual life. It certainly has an important place in many of the world's great religions, whether one is en route to Mecca, Santiago di Compostella or Bodh Gaya. In India today many families will combine pilgrimage with their annual holidays, with the extended family travelling together to sacred places, temples, churches and mosques across the length and breadth of the subcontinent.

The atmosphere created at these gatherings can be profoundly transformative, to say the least. In 1998 I went on a pilgrimage to the sacred hill of Arunachala in South India, arriving at midnight on the last day of the ten-day festival known as Kartigai Deepam. Over the following 24 hours, a million people arrived in the small town of Tiruvannamalai situated at the base of the hill. Many thousands of them walked barefoot up the 700-metre hill to witness the lighting of a huge vessel of ghee at the moment of sunset on that day.

The light from the huge fire can be seen for many miles in the surrounding countryside and at the exact moment it is lit, local villagers and townsfolk will light small candles throughout their homes. The deepam or lamp symbolically represents the spiritual light of understanding of the true nature of reality and it has been lit in such fashion over many thousands of years.

What I remember most vividly was the tremendous feeling of camaraderie among the pilgrims as we climbed the hill. They came from all walks of life, many having travelled hundreds of kilometres to get there. The level of concern for the wellbeing of the assembled walkers was truly touching and there was a shared feeling of elation at being part of this ancient tradition.

PILGRIMAGE IS, BY ITS NATURE, A VERY PERSONAL EXPERIENCE …

At the end of the day, having completed the trek, I found myself having a meal with five new Indian friends. There was a lovely ease of conversation among us and an open sharing of the situations that life had placed us in. There seemed to be an unspoken but heartfelt appreciation of the spirit that animates us all.

Pilgrimage is, by its nature, a very personal experience and may take many different forms depending on the person. In essence it is a journey that is about something larger than your selfish needs and desires; it is a calling to your heart and sometimes it will not make much sense to your rational mind. There may be an intuition that it is something that just needs to be done.

My own journey to Uluru in central Australia was certainly made in that spirit. As someone born in Australia, it seemed somehow important to have an experience of this sacred place and to linger there for a while. Needless to say, my four-hour walk around the rock had a deep impact on me, which I am still digesting to this day. I felt as if I was beholding the most extraordinary piece of modern sculpture on the planet – its dimensions, form, colour and texture transporting me to another dimension, far removed from the usual landscapes of my mind.

A pilgrim's masala

I include this account from a colleague of mine who travelled to India on her own as a young woman in the 1990s. Reading her words, it is easy to get a sense of the many dimensions of the experience of pilgrimage and the learning that can come with that experience. For those not versed in Indian cooking, a masala is a spice mix.

I had been gorging myself on the wisdom teachings of India for years before I finally made the pilgrimage to the motherland. I was warned to make a good itinerary before going and to throw it out the window upon arrival – the best travel advice ever! Suffice to say my visit was a bit like a full-frontal spiritual practice, marked by many little pilgrimages – a few intentional ones and the rest by divine accident.

As with any worthwhile experience, surrender is the key. It opens the gates to the holy ground where transformation can take place. For example, if you resist the fullness of India's flavour, you end up on an auto-rickshaw being ushered through the nearest Indian emporium. If you relax and let the sensory overload take you where it will, India will reveal the most unlikely places where its most precious jewels are to be found. My first lesson in surrender came straight off the tarmac in India, when I entered a taxi only to face Jesus on the dashboard in flashing lights – what was He doing in Cochin! Lesson two – risking malaria is preferable to sucking in a precariously hung mosquito net every night! Lesson three – most Brahmin priests in landmark temples are praying on your purse ... And so on. Each encounter was a subtle chiselling away at expectation until I gave up having any and just went with the flow.

This process of undoing is mirrored in temple etiquette, which requires you to propitiate the elephant-headed god Ganesh first, before making your way into the rest of the temple. Locals tell you it is to prevent him from making mischief while you are in there. However, as the remover of obstacles, he represents the all-important act of emptying out, leaving your baggage and your preconceptions at the door, once again, to create the space for transformation.

Reverence is a vital ingredient to add to the pilgrim's masala. Without reverence, a pilgrimage becomes a tourist destination. It is the fuel and compass for the journey. Without some form of reverence for India, I might have been put off, as many are, at the first sight of extreme poverty. I might have cursed the screeching monkeys at Sri Ramanashramam and missed the deeper sentiment of peace that permeated the place. I might have had a panic attack when a public bus dropped me in the middle of Tamil Nadu with dirt roads forking off in opposite directions and local folks insisting that both directions were the correct way to the Abhirami Temple. Reverence is like the heart's song and it calls in the experiences you need.

Awareness, or the ability to listen for the divine timing of things and act intuitively, is another main ingredient. India has a remarkable way of heightening your awareness. I think that because many of the experiences there are so foreign to the comparatively sedate pace in Australia, and also because your cognitive mind and senses are bombarded with so many stimuli, you are forced over into your right brain to cope.

During my visit to India I made many intentional pilgrimages to yoga centres and temples that I had heard about, but my most treasured experience was one that unfolded out of a series of fortuitous encounters with strangers. They included an old doctor of Siddha medicine on a midnight bus ride in Tamil Nadu, an Ayurvedic patient I made friends with at Poonthotham Ayurveda Hospital in Kerala and then ran into on the east coast, and a close relative of Arthur Osborne, who founded the Mountain Path *magazines at the ashram dedicated to Sri Ramana Maharishi. If I hadn't been following my heart (because I had thrown my itinerary out the window), I wouldn't have gone on the winding path that led me to Sri Ramanashramam and the cave where the great saint Ramana Maharishi had lived in silence.*

Respect is another essential ingredient. It's impossible not to be in awe of the spiritual teachers who have blazed the trail and signposted some of the important landmarks that are common to a spiritual path. But when you physically make a pilgrimage to places that have a spiritual potency about them, respect is inevitable and you find yourself overcome, humbled and usually speechless ... for a while, at least.

The place of spiritual retreat

Another way to support your spiritual practice is to remove yourself from your working and family life and spend some time in a retreat centre or ashram. This experience offers the possibility of a deeper level of introspection than when you are caught up in the distractions and responsibilities of working and family life. It can offer you some mental space and time to digest both positive and negative life experiences in a safe and supportive environment.

Spiritual retreats allow you to be part of a daily program that may involve gentle yoga exercises in the morning, periods of meditation and the opportunity to practise selfless work. A morning of Karma yoga may involve gardening, food preparation or cleaning and provides you with the opportunity to integrate spiritual teachings into daily life. It can also be an opportunity to meet like-minded people who may at some stage become part of your own spiritual community.

While staying at an ashram in India, I had a breakthrough with an issue that had plagued me in my early adult life. The issue was cleaning – specifically, cleaning toilets. This was something I had been spared during my adolescent years thanks to my mother and the fact that we had professional cleaners coming to our family home on a regular basis. The net result was that I had never developed a habit around household cleaning and this had become a source of tension for housemates I had shared with over the years.

During my month in the ashram, I was given the role of cleaning the toilets each morning as my Karma yoga. As there were over ten toilets in the block in which I was living, I soon became adept at the task. The happy outcome of this work is that I am now much more aware of the need for bathroom cleanliness and will, of my own volition, clean the toilet reasonably frequently and with a fair degree of diligence in my own home. An unexpected boon born of the retreat experience!

Most retreat centres discourage the taking of recreational drugs, cigarettes, coffee and alcohol, so you can use the time to detoxify for a few days. They also discourage or prohibit the use of computers, radio and television, as they are seen as scattering your thought processes and keeping your mind at a more superficial level.

Many retreat centres are located in beautiful natural settings that support relaxation of body and mind and tend to ground the busy, overstimulated mind that most of us experience a lot of the time. Just being there, even without doing

117

any practices, can bring profound transformative experiences and epiphanies, as you benefit from the collective intention and energy of others at the retreat.

During your time at the retreat, you can learn about practices that encourage body–mind integration including yoga postures, breathing exercises and different techniques of meditation. The practice of these and the conditions provided at the centre promote deeper experiences in meditation and the insights into oneself that often come with that. These in turn can support a change in your basic perception of yourself and others and lay the foundation for a different way of being in the world.

The role of practice

Without doubt the most important aspect of spiritual practice is the act of practising. When you commit to a daily practice, this itself brings its own rewards. You know that, no matter what kind of drama or uncertainty is unfolding in your life, your spiritual practice will continue. In this way it becomes a central platform in your daily life; something that doesn't change even though the outward expression of your life might. The actual practice of your sadhana helps to create an inner strength and resilience, and something that you can call upon when the going gets tough.

For many people, the reading of spiritual literature is a powerful and immediate way to nourish your spiritual practice. Spiritual literature affirms your intuition, elevates your mood or brings a measure of stillness to your mind. The life stories and autobiographies of saints are especially recommended as sources of inspiration. As one revered elderly teacher of yoga pointed out in a public talk in Sydney many years ago, the fact that you may not be able to emulate the feats of such beings is not important. Like the stars in the night sky, you know that you will never reach them, but their very presence calls you forth and opens you to something greater than your present, preoccupying concerns.

Bringing spiritual practice into my everyday life

Melissa has combined a career in law, marriage celebrancy and teaching yoga with being a single parent. Here she shares how spiritual practice has impacted on her life.

My personal sadhana or spiritual practice has underpinned and upheld my sanity as a single mum, soothed my soul, strengthened my resolve and provided peace. It has varied over the years.

For me, what works is giving the gift of peace to myself first thing in the morning, filling up my cup the better to fill or help others fill theirs. Daily or regular meditation or at least a period in the day for quiet self-reflection is the key. It may just be waking up, lighting a candle and a stick of incense and sitting in a special quiet space.

For many years, yoga has been a tool for mental and physical purification and spiritual nourishment. More recently, after 22 years I have rediscovered Vipassana meditation as taught by Goenka. This has been of tremendous help to me in all areas of life.

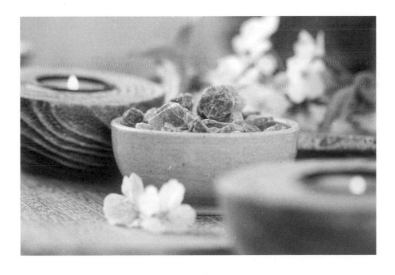

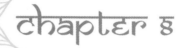

Chapter 8

Finding your path

In order to lead a meaningful life, you need to cherish others, pay attention to human values and try to cultivate inner peace.

The 14th Dalai Lama

Early in my medical career, prior to studying Ayurveda, a young man in his early twenties was referred to me with mild depression. When I met Joshua, I could see a dark cloud of negative thoughts hanging over him that no doubt was contributing to his low mood. His father had died a year previously and when I saw him, Joshua was working as a clerk in a large accounting firm, a job he hated. Not surprisingly he had developed a cynical attitude to life. The GP who had referred Joshua to me felt that he would benefit from learning meditation, which I was incorporating in my medical practice with selected patients.

Joshua took to the practice of meditation easily and experienced times when he felt more positive and even peaceful. During our talks it emerged that his real passion in life was acting, which he had enjoyed and excelled at in high school. However, his mother had strongly discouraged him from following a career in acting, which in her view was a financially unreliable and difficult way to make a living.

I suggested that there was no harm in at least applying to a number of drama schools around the country, which he did. Several months later, Joshua was accepted into one of the most prestigious acting courses in Australia and later moved interstate to take up his place.

Over the next few years I lost touch with Joshua, and when I did see him again in the waiting room of my medical practice, I could barely recognise him. His demeanour, posture and bearing had totally changed. He exuded a confidence and enthusiasm that was palpable. Now working in a well-known acting company, he was currently performing in a Shakespearian comedy and was obviously thriving in the creative milieu that acting provided for him. I had a strong sense that Joshua was doing what he was meant to be doing at that time in his life. More than that, it was clear he had found his path.

In this chapter I explore the idea that there is a path through life for all of us as individuals which is fundamentally supportive of our physical, emotional, mental and spiritual wellbeing. As each of us is part of a complex matrix that includes our friends, families and communities, this path brings considerable benefits for them as well. In Ayurveda, that path is known as your dharma.

Your personal dharma

The concept of dharma is a foundation stone of the civilisation of the subcontinent of India. Like many words in Sanskrit, the language of ancient India, it has a number of different meanings. At the cosmic level it refers to the inherent laws of nature that sustain the operation of the universe. At the level of the individual, it is the path through life that allows you to live to your full potential: the path that best fits your individual nature, including your temperament, aptitudes and talents, in the context of the family and society into which you were born.

Certainly, dharma is a complex concept and it has been interpreted in various ways through the ages. The word 'dharma' is derived from the root dhar, meaning 'to hold, maintain or preserve'. It refers to those things in life that support us as we journey through life; activities that keep us grounded, healthy and connected into the bigger picture. Traditionally in India it is taken to refer to the performance of duties and rituals that are an expected part of Hindu life.

In essence, your personal dharma is a calling to honour and actualise your uniqueness as a human being. It is not a selfish endeavour, but rather something that will carry you through life in a way that produces a sense of deep satisfaction. Honouring your dharma may involve doing things that are boring, inconvenient or unpleasant at times, but when those things are in the service of your dharma, they are accepted quite naturally.

World champion surfer and surfing pioneer, Wayne Lynch, puts it well:

> *If you follow your own heart you will find that you've lived the life you're meant to be living, no matter what hardships or ridicule or whatever happens. It won't be a perfect life, it won't be an easy life, but it's your life and you'll feel really good about that life.*

Many people describe a knowing that comes to them when they are doing something in line with their dharma. A knowing that says, 'This is what I am meant to be doing on the planet at this moment.'

Carl Jung, the visionary Swiss psychiatrist and thinker, writing in the early part of the 20th century, coined the term 'individuation', which he described as living into your wholeness as a human being. Abraham Maslow, an American pioneer in the human growth movement in the latter part of the 20th century, talked about 'self-actualisation', which is when a person is living into their highest potential. Both of these terms are helpful in giving us a sense of the meaning of personal dharma.

Importantly the concept of dharma recognises that human beings are social creatures and part of an intricate web of relationships. As you journey through life, you take on many roles: as a son or daughter, as a sibling, as a friend, as a partner, as a workmate and as a parent. It encourages us to be mindful of our responsibilities and to honour these relationships in practical ways. By standing up for a younger sibling in a high school setting, by honouring your partner's needs for time and space and by taking the time to visit an aged parent in a nursing home, we honour our personal dharma. In this sense respect for the other, as a basis for relationship, is central to connecting with your dharma. It is a respect that also requires us to develop a capacity for self-sacrifice, when living our dharma.

The metaphor of a tapestry is helpful in understanding dharma. If you are a single thread in the overall tapestry of life, the tapestry supports you. But the integrity of the tapestry is only as strong as the strength and integrity of each individual thread. So the tapestry supports you and you support the tapestry;

you are dependent on each other. When you live fully in your different roles in life, mindful of your duties, everyone benefits – your friends, your family, your community, your country and the planet as a whole.

In this way connecting with your personal dharma can become a pathway to a fulfilling life. Following a purely selfish personal agenda brings short-lived pleasure, whereas when we express ourselves authentically and in a way that honours other sentient beings and Mother Earth, a more enduring satisfaction arises.

An important aspect of your personal dharma is your livelihood. Ideally it's the kind of activity that allows you to express yourself authentically in the workplace, in the home and in your community, whether as a businessperson, stay-at-home parent or as a caregiver to an elderly relative.

While living and studying Ayurveda at a university in Gujarat in India, I was lodged in a postgraduate men's hostel. Each morning, the sweeper would knock on my door and ask if he could come in and sweep my room. One morning, when my room was in a particularly messy state, I told him not to bother that day. He replied, 'But sir, it is my duty.' It took me a while to realise what he was expressing and to appreciate that he needed to be able to perform this task that was his responsibility; a responsibility he took seriously.

When you are living in line with your dharma, whatever that might be, there are profound benefits for your physical and mental health. Your life force or prana, as it is known in yoga, is significantly stronger and it becomes much harder to get sick. Through living more in the flow of life, your personal energy gets nourished and replenished in an ongoing way. You are then better placed to be there for your partner, family, workmates and the people you encounter through the day. By making a positive difference to their world in some way, you get to feel good about yourself and your endeavours. In this way connecting with your dharma is inherently good for your self-esteem and sense of self-worth.

Connecting with my dharma

The movement into alignment with your dharma is well illustrated by the experiences of Stephanie, a graphic designer and reflexologist (practitioner of foot massage), who went back to her childhood to find inspiration and renewal.

The constant niggle of wanting a career change and an urge to investigate a more meaningful and purposeful life began when I was feeling disconnected and uninterested in my job. My main interaction was with a computer, tight deadlines and stressed-out work colleagues. My work was rushed and churned out. I had an overwhelming sense that I had more to offer the world.

I began to receive counselling about areas in which I felt stuck – work being the major one. In one session my counsellor gave me homework to make a visual board of my life desires. I creatively set about cutting out pictures and words from magazines and newspapers. My intent and focus was also on past experiences that brought me joy and a sense of effortless action.

I reflected on times in my childhood when Mum would lovingly massage my feet after I played representative netball all weekend. My feet would be tired and aching. I lay blissfully and receptively on the couch and would disappear into a deep and restorative sleep. On waking I was filled with a profound sense of relaxation. It was as though I had been suspended in time and space – my whole being held peacefully in her hands.

When I went back to my next counselling session – board in hand – it was curiously pointed out that I had a lot of pictures with feet in them. Reflexology was talked about as a possible path to investigate. A new connection was revealing itself to me … feet.

I set about researching reflexology, as it had never been on my radar before. The mind, body and soul connection had always been of interest to me though. The gift from my mother had planted a seed in me and it was now being unearthed! I booked myself into a weekend workshop to see if this tactile and healing therapy was meant for me. I was hooked! When I was massaging a person's foot it felt as though I was a musician playing an instrument. There was a definite rhythm and joy that came from giving someone a treatment. I found my zone. Then my path from weekend course to practitioner was seamless. My new direction felt like I had a purpose and that it was destined, rather than choosing a new career.

When seeking my life purpose or dharma it was necessary to make a commitment to myself – both in mind and body. I chose to tackle the journey from a creative angle, which gave me different and important perspectives. It was the visual cue that ignited the enquiry.

My dharma required counselling, reflection, dedicated work, consistent effort, a strength to go my own way and practising on as many feet that I could lay my hands on! I also stayed open to the coincidences that came my way, the new people I was meeting from reflexology and the opportunities that the universe presented to me.

Seeds may lay dormant for many years as to your purpose, but when they are unearthed there is powerful growth and a new determined energy that springs from within.

Trust that there is a path for you, that is continually unfolding. And practise, practise, practise …

Finding your personal dharma

In traditional Indian culture Vedic astrology is used as an aid to help individuals connect with the path through life that will best support them. By looking at the areas of your birth chart specifically related to your dharma, as well as through analysis of the general tenor of your birth chart, a good astrologer can suggest the sort of vocation that you may be best suited to.

In a contemporary Western context, Western astrology can also be a powerful aid in getting some direction with your dharma, as we shall see later in this chapter. Specifically, we will explore how your astrological birth chart can be an invaluable tool for personal guidance and help you live into your full potential.

Your intuitive leanings, as impractical as they might seem at the time, can also be profoundly accurate in the process of connecting with your dharma. At times there may not be great clarity about what it is you are meant to be doing with your life, but rather a vague sense of the direction to be followed. This is where the role of synchronicity or meaningful coincidences can also have a powerful bearing on how your dharma unfolds. Your intuition can serve you well in your journey through life, and I'll return to this important theme shortly.

It is also true that for some people, finding their personal dharma can be a lengthy process. Not everyone knows at the age of twelve that they want to be a writer and then steadfastly follows that dream. Often there are many twists, turns and a few blind alleys along the way. Trial and error may be a necessary part of getting more clarity and an important vehicle for growth and learning. In this sense, connecting with your dharma could best be described as a process of refinement throughout your life.

For lots of us, connecting with a unifying sense of purpose in terms of how to expend your energy each day can be very challenging. This is especially the case when there is not a lot of family or other support to follow the callings of your heart. Commonly, you will have to contend with a parental agenda, loving or not so loving, of how your life should turn out. Needless to say, this can result in a lot of conflict and tension in the parent–child relationship, which itself needs to be managed.

Health tip

When we connect with our dharma, our prana (life force) becomes stronger and it is harder to get sick.

Connecting with your dharma can require a lot of courage. I am reminded of an old friend of mine who was born into a family of conservative southern European immigrants who came to Australia after World War II. On finishing school, Maria was expected to stay at home for the rest of her life and look after her parents in their old age. Despite the fact that she was dux of her school there was no question of her leaving home, let alone pursuing further study at university. In fact when she did decide to leave home her father didn't speak to her for five years. To her enormous credit, Maria followed her love of painting and studied at a college of fine arts, later marrying another painter and having two delightful children.

Tapping into your inner knowing

The intuitive mind is a sacred gift and the rational mind is a faithful servant.
We have created a society that honours the servant and has forgotten the gift.

Albert Einstein

One of the things that attracted me to the ancient healing traditions of India was the central place given to subjective experience. Meditation, in its various forms, is seen as a means to penetrate into the depths of human experience and is fundamental for the development of self-knowledge and self-healing. Central to the importance given to meditation is the idea that within all of us is an incredibly wise being with access to timeless knowledge and understanding. Knowledge and understanding that is specifically tailored to our unique needs and which has our best interests at heart.

When we are able to connect with that still place that exists inside all of us all the time, the part of us that is timeless and changeless, we make ourselves more receptive to its subtle messages. In the words of Sri Ramana Maharshi, a revered south Indian spiritual teacher who lived during the 20th century: 'Silence is ever-speaking; it is the perennial flow of language; it is interrupted by speaking. These words obstruct that mute language.'

The idea that stillness and silence are full of potentiality has been a fundamental tenet of the spiritual tradition of yoga for thousands of years.

When you are able to tap into your inner knowing there are enormous practical benefits. You may be struggling with questions such as: 'Is this the right house to buy? Will this job suit my needs? Should I be entering into a committed relationship with this person? Is the food I am about to eat best suited for my body type?' By developing your intuitive faculty you can support your mental and physical wellbeing in undreamt of ways.

The importance of the intuitive realm was well recognised by the Swiss psychologist Carl Jung who articulated the various ways in which the soul communicates with us in order to help us live to our fullest potential. Some of the ways that the soul 'whispers' to us include: synchronicities or meaningful coincidences, dreams, bodily symptoms, mishaps and chronic illness.

By contrast, the mainstream approach to learning in the West focuses largely on the use of the rational mind. In order to understand something or to work through a problem, we are taught to use our intellect and through a process that uses analysis, logic and reasoning gain insights into the subject being investigated. There is no doubt that this is a powerful and practical approach to gaining knowledge and one that has been embraced by humanity throughout the ages to enormous benefit.

But it is also true that there are other ways to gain knowledge and understanding of the world; ways that cultivate a relationship with the intuitive realm. We can see this principle clearly at work in the shamanic traditions of indigenous cultures the world over where information that comes through non-rational channels is highly valued and sought after. The Tibetan government has for centuries, as well as presently, used the services of a state oracle whose utterances in the context of a complex spiritual ritual influence the formulation of that government's policies.

Many of the greatest discoveries in Western science have involved non-linear thought processes. Indeed Einstein's conceptual leap in his work on quantum physics came to him as if in a dream, when he saw himself riding on a beam of light. He concluded that if he were to do so, light would appear static. This led him to the concept of relativity, which fundamentally changed physics and how we understand the workings of the universe.

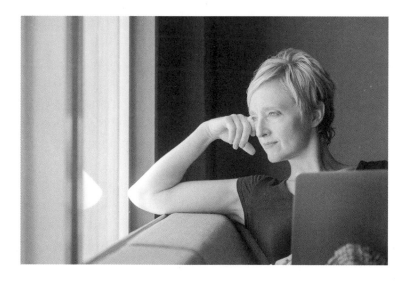

Supporting your intuition

Ayurveda sees intuition as a God-given gift and part of your birthright as a human being. But what do we mean by intuition? It's a word that gets thrown around a lot in common language. The *Oxford English Dictionary* defines intuition as 'the immediate apprehension of an object by the mind without the intervention of any reasoning process'. Over the last fifteen years, I have asked hundreds of students, mostly women I might add, this same question. Speaking from their own experience, they have described the hallmarks of intuitive experience, saying it is not a cognitive process and does not involve past experience. For some it is a visceral experience that is felt in the body; others simply describe it as a knowing. They describe it as knowledge that comes to you, that is not sought. Many say that it is knowledge that can help you in some way, even though how it will help may not be clear at the time the intuitive insight arises.

There are many ways to support your intuition and develop a more lively and close relationship with it. For a start, you can consciously invite the intuitive dimension into your life and allow it to flower in its own way. Many of the practices of yoga, meditation and Ayurveda are inherently supportive of your intuition.

When practised regularly, yoga postures appropriate to your age and health, make the body more vital and energetic. As you begin to inhabit your body more fully and connect with your legs and feet, you begin to connect with the energies of the earth. You learn how to stay grounded and more present to the unfolding moment and any whispers coming from the intuitive realm.

The practice of meditation, particularly meditation practices that encourage connection with the body, can also help support your intuition. For many people, learning to enjoy your own company and quiet time can be a major challenge. This is where learning a specific meditation practice from a teacher you respect can be immensely useful. You learn how to rest into the moment and connect with your five senses, rather than getting caught up in the content of your thoughts.

Spending time in nature is another great way to support your intuition. When you tune into the energies of your back garden, the ocean or a forest, you quite naturally open to the intuitive dimension. Watching the movement of waves, listening to the subtle rustling sound of leaves and smelling the scents of the flowers can transport you to very different realms of experience in a short space of time.

Developing a more attentive relationship with your dreams is another simple way to support your intuitive faculty. Keeping a dream journal or simply writing down or drawing dreams that seem somehow significant to you is a helpful practice and encourages a different kind of receptivity in your being. Allowing yourself to lie in bed and passively contemplate a dream you have had the night before is another way to open up to information from this other realm.

Being around people who are more tuned into their intuition can make a big difference to your ability to listen to and trust your intuition. It is very easy for people who pride themselves on their rationality to dismiss the experience of others who are following a gut feeling or a position that is not backed up by a solid reason. By contrast, people who are more in touch with their right brain function are likely to be interested in your seemingly random experiences.

As you begin to tune into the intuitive realm and what it has to say to you, you can then start to act on the guidance it is giving. Taking on a spirit of naive experimentation in relation to intuitive messages is a useful approach. You can then begin to see for yourself whether the information coming to you has some kind of utility in your life or not. As you start to trust your intuition, it can become a most valuable resource and help you in making choices that support your health and wellbeing.

What your intuition is saying may be at odds with what your rational mind is thinking about the matter at hand, though it is also possible that the two approaches can be in accord and can support each other.

 ## How intuition has helped in my life

The practical use of intuition in daily life is well illustrated by the experiences of a colleague of mine. Nina, a single parent, natural therapist and yoga teacher shares how intuition operates in her life and how it helps her in unexpected ways.

My personal experience of intuition is as an inner guidance system, and a sense of knowing, often beyond my conscious understanding. I guess it's a bit like having a mental filter that helps me discern the most useful opportunities and life experiences.

Throughout my life I've experienced intuition in a few different ways: as a sense of rightness and of being led, an inexplicable knowing, a feeling of stirring or aligning, a sense of imminent change or that something has been set in motion, and 'I'm on the right track'. I may feel a heightened sensory awareness, and my surroundings may seem crisper and colours brighter than usual.

When I tune in, my life seems to run more smoothly. So when making decisions, I take notice of those feelings of knowing and of any resistance in my body; that 'it just doesn't feel right' feeling. I believe that the right things can happen easily, without forcing or feeling like you're going against the grain. There is a big difference between positive persistence and forcing, and forcing just doesn't seem to work out well.

Recently I was presented with a business opportunity that ticked a lot of the boxes in terms of how it fitted in with my values and family life. But whenever I thought about it, I felt resistance. A kind of contraction in my body. It felt as if things wouldn't flow well with this business, it just didn't sit right. So I didn't go ahead with it and I felt the relief and ease of letting that one go.

I try to connect with my intuitive sense when reflecting on my health and physical needs by turning inwards and noticing sensations, feelings and thoughts that arise. At times I may receive a specific instruction such as eat a certain food or a drive to have a particular kind of treatment, or there may be themes that arise such as rest, energise, movement.

In work situations as a natural therapist, I sometimes experience a strong sense of a client even before the consultation; a sense of the important themes or issues the person is dealing with and the remedy or treatment that would be useful for them. It may be a spontaneous word or phrase (as in clairaudience), or a feeling evoked from their body language. I consider this the kind of intuition built from years of experience as a therapist, intuition that draws on my subconscious and the experience of archetypes.

Astrology: Having Mother Nature on your side

We are born at a given moment in a given place and like vintage years of wine we have the qualities of the year and of the season in which we are born. Astrology does not lay claim to anything else.

Carl Jung

Here in the West, astrology is generally viewed with a high degree of scepticism mixed with humour. It is the stuff of magazines and newspaper columns, often written by non-astrologers, full of generalisations and the promise of tall, dark strangers about to walk into your life and change things forever.

Despite this, most people will know something about their star sign and many will tell you that they can relate to a lot of the traits associated with it. In an age where the rational approach of science is the dominant paradigm, astrology is not to be taken seriously. Moreover, Judeo-Christian religious traditions have actively outlawed astrology for hundreds of years and seen it as the devil's work; an aspect of the occult world you play with at your peril.

By contrast, the ancient world has a tremendous feeling for and interest in the celestial realms and their relationship with our physical world. During my time living and studying in India, I encountered a radically different relationship with astrology in society at large. In India, astrologers are held in high regard by the general population and are consulted freely on all sorts of matters. When a child is born, someone in the family will be charged with the responsibility of recording the exact moment of birth, so that an accurate birth chart can be drawn up. When a prospective marriage partner is found, one of the first things to be done by the parents is to engage a trusted family astrologer, to see whether that person's birth chart will be a good match for their son or daughter. The most auspicious time to start a business or the building of a dwelling will often involve consulting an astrologer in an effort to align with the cycles of the sun, moon, planets and stars.

Vedic astrology, known in India as Jyotish, is one of the fundamental building blocks of traditional Indian society and is still very much used in contemporary

Indian life. While it has important differences with Western astrology, there are also a number of significant similarities. It is a sister science of Ayurveda and yoga, informing and complementing both. In the following sections I focus on how knowledge of your astrological birth chart can be an extremely useful guide in the art of balanced living.

The wisdom traditions of India acknowledge the unity of all life; we are all part of an extraordinarily complex web. One of the defining features of a spider's web is that if you pull on one part of the web, the rest of the web is necessarily affected in some way, whether strongly or subtly. In the same way, we human beings are connected through a complex system of relationships with the rest of the universe.

These relationships extend into the physical world, including other human beings, animals, plants, landforms and climates. The microcosm of the human body is seen as being in a state of ongoing interaction with the macrocosm of the outside world. This understanding necessarily includes the celestial bodies and as such looks to see how they influence the behaviour of human beings and the world at large.

The birth chart for an individual is a representation of the specific astronomical pattern at the time and place of your birth. It records where the sun, moon and planets were in the sky relative to the constellations of the stars at the specific time and place that you first appeared on the earth.

Health tip

Having an understanding of your child's birth chart can be invaluable in appreciating how they are different to you.

In order to construct a birth chart, the date, time and place of birth of the individual is required. In Western astrology, a circular chart is drawn up that is essentially a map of the heavens at the moment of that person's birth. This circle is divided twelve times corresponding to the twelve signs of the zodiac, or 'wheel of animals', as it was noted in ancient times that some of the constellations looked like animals or symbols. On top of this circle is superimposed twelve pie-shaped divisions known as houses. These houses relate to areas of life experience, both in outer day-to-day life and inner, psychological life.

Areas of life represented by the twelve houses

First house	Physical appearance, body type and how you take action
Second house	What you value in life, material resources, especially money, and your sense of self-worth
Third house	Communication style, schooling and siblings
Fourth house	Your home, family life and childhood experiences
Fifth house	Creative expression, children and love affairs
Sixth house	Your health, daily work and rituals
Seventh house	Marriage and partnerships
Eighth house	Sexuality, death and the occult
Ninth house	Higher education, travel and approach to religion
Tenth house	Career, vocation and attitude to authority
Eleventh house	Participation in groups and social reform
Twelfth house	Involvement in institutions such as hospitals, prisons and schools and past life actions

Birth chart showing placement of sun, moon and ascendant

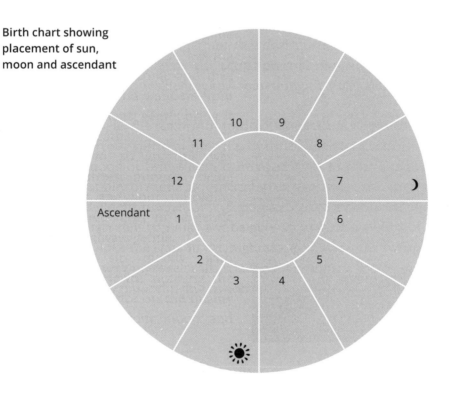

In essence, the birth chart is like a blueprint for your journey in this lifetime. Being a dynamic principle that changes in accordance with the cycles of the sun, moon, planets and the constellations, it is a system for understanding how those energies will unfold in time and how they are likely to influence you. In this context your birth chart, when properly understood, can become a valuable tool to help you realise your full potential as a human being.

Reading your birth chart

By studying your individual birth chart, a competent astrologer will have access to information about many different aspects of your life. Through an understanding of the interaction between the energies of the sun, moon and planets, set against the twelve constellations of stars and superimposed on the twelve houses, the astrologer gets an idea of strengths and challenges inherent in the birth chart of the person coming for the consultation.

In Western astrology, your star sign is determined by which of the twelve specific constellations that appear to circle the Earth forms the backdrop for the sun when viewed from your birthplace at the time and date of your birth. The twelve signs of the zodiac, moving from Aries through to Pisces, correspond with these twelve specific constellations.

The sign in which your sun is placed, what is commonly called your star sign, relates to your core identity; who you are in essence and what drives you. For example, someone born with their sun in Cancer, unless this is overridden by other factors in their chart, has an inherent need to nurture and protect those they consider to be family.

By contrast, someone born with a sun sign in Libra may have an inherent need to find balance and harmony in their life. In this sense, they may be natural mediators, well able to utilise their negotiation skills to resolve conflict.

The sign (or constellation) in which the moon is placed relates to your instinctive nature and your unconscious. It tells the Western astrologer about what makes you feel nurtured. Someone with their moon in Taurus is likely to feel nurtured by sensuality – food, music and massage. By contrast, someone with their moon placed in Gemini may feel more nurtured by new ideas and systems of thought.

The ascendant, or rising sign, is the sign of the zodiac that was ascending or rising on the eastern horizon at the time of your birth. It is an important part of your personality and relates to the persona or mask that you present to the world. Someone with a rising sign in Aries will tend to come across in an assertive and direct way. They are doers who take initiative easily. Whereas someone with a rising sign in Aquarius is more likely to be experienced as very individualistic and even quirky on first meeting.

In this way, the sun, moon and ascendant are important points of reference in understanding the birth chart and much can be gleaned about the nature of the person coming for a reading from these three primary energies. The placement of the planets relative to the constellations, moving from Mercury, which is closest to the sun, through to Pluto, which is furthest from the sun, adds another layer of complexity and further scope for understanding the nature of the individual.

THE ACCURATE READING OF THE BIRTH CHART ... IS BEST DESCRIBED AS AN ART FORM.

Each of the planets is associated with a specific archetype having a set of qualities or drives that define it. An archetype is an innate, universal pattern of thought or an image present in the human psyche. The archetype of Mars represents the desire for action and the courage to fight for what we want. The archetype of Venus represents our personal values, our urge for pleasure and how we attract others into our lives. The archetype of Saturn relates to our ability to organise our lives and take responsibility. Our personal boundaries and the power to discipline ourselves are under the influence of Saturn.

The accurate reading of the birth chart, as you may be gathering, is an extremely complex process requiring proper training and a great deal of experience. It is best described as an art form. A further exposition of the basic tenets of astrology is beyond the scope of this book and I refer readers interested in knowing more about both Western and Vedic astrology to the Further Reading section at the end of this book.

The birth chart as a tool for personal guidance

When understood as a blueprint for your journey in this lifetime, your birth chart can be a powerful aid in helping you live into your full potential. The astrologer may be seeing the blueprint of a 26-room mansion with water views, only to find you are living in the basement. The astrologer's job therefore is to help the client realise the full expression of their individual nature; in Ayurvedic terminology, to align with their personal dharma.

This will entail an analysis of the natural gifts of that person, as well as identifying any limiting tendencies that may need to be resolved in order for them to find fulfilment and success. Often people take for granted some of their innate talents.

When an individual is going through a tough time, the astrologer is well placed to see why those difficulties may be arising. The underlying reason for the difficulty may be a limiting belief system or a challenging personal situation or a combination of both. The astrologer can then help the client navigate that difficulty by mobilising the resources they do possess or through suggesting some kind of remedial measure or referral to an appropriate agency.

Health tip

An insightful reading of your birth chart can help you navigate the challenges of life.

For example, the person coming for an astrological consultation may be going through a period of marital disharmony. This may be related to difficulties in how they communicate, some aspect of their personality, or their choice of partner. The difficulties may be exacerbated by workplace stress and/or financial worries. Through a thorough analysis of the person's birth chart, the astrologer can shed light on the root causes of the disharmony. The astrologer can then recommend any number of measures, from receiving individual or couples counselling, to learning better techniques for managing stress or finding ways to communicate more effectively, in order to support the client.

As mentioned previously, Vedic astrology is often used to help people get a sense of where their vocation in life might lie. Through studying the parts of the birth chart specifically related to an individual's livelihood in the context of their chart as a whole, a good astrologer is able to suggest the sort of vocation and work that that person is best suited to. Here the astrologer is making an assessment of the strengths and challenges inherent in the person's chart, and the kind of work that is most likely to marry with those qualities.

To illustrate this point, I share with you an experience I had many years ago during a consultation with Hart De Fouw, a Western adept in Vedic astrology. I consulted Hart for a general reading of my birth chart, as someone interested in self-knowledge and the unique perspectives that this tradition might offer. During the reading he asked me if I had any interest in writing. To which I replied, 'Not really.' 'Why is that?' he enquired. 'Well, to my mind all the great books have already been written, people just need to read them.' To which he countered, 'Well, that may be true, but I would like to suggest two things to you. Firstly, knowledge needs to be renewed through the writing of new books; and secondly, if writing figures significantly in your birth chart, not to write is to do yourself and your community a disservice.'

His comments, born from an analysis of my birth chart, challenged my accepted thinking on the subject of writing and my relationship with it. I started to see the wisdom of his words and later came to embrace the place of writing in my vision for myself. At high school, English had been a subject I had excelled in, but I hadn't explored it further during my time in medical school. As a result of Hart's reading, my attitude to writing underwent a significant transformation. This culminated in the publishing of my first book in 2003, a decade after his reading. Over the past 20 years I have written many pieces for textbooks, magazines and blogs, which has been very helpful in the promotion of my medical practice and in my work as an educator.

Hart had seen something in my chart that needed to find expression, which would be important in my growth and development as a human being. Certainly from my perspective, I can see that as someone keen to contribute to the intellectual discourse of the age I have been born into, writing was always going to be an important aspect of my self-expression. It remains to be seen whether I would ever have become a published author if not for Hart's presence and his gentle confrontation all those years ago.

Your unfolding birth chart

Your birth chart represents a snapshot of the heavens at the moment that you first appeared on planet Earth. From that moment the sun, moon, planets and stars move in their own specific cycles in an ongoing fashion. This necessarily creates a changing set of relationships between these celestial bodies that influence the birth chart. Specific parts of the chart are highlighted at certain times, so to speak, and accordingly those areas of your life will be given more energy and become more active.

In this way, an astrology reading can give you information about the themes that may lie ahead for you in the coming months or years. This can be extremely useful in allowing you to prepare, both mentally and physically, for future events that may transpire. For example, the astrologer may see the likelihood of a child being conceived or a period where you need to be vigilant about your health or the possibility of upcoming financial challenges. Forewarned is forearmed and the awareness coming from the reading can help you better navigate the likely territory in front of you.

Just as an expert botanist can tell the difference between an apple seed and the seed of an orange, and is fully conversant with the differences between the fully grown trees, a good astrologer can see the potential in a person's birth chart. They may well be able to see something currently hidden from the client, something that with some encouragement may help the client to live into their fullness. If the client is young and lacking in confidence, by validating the talents of that person clearly seen in the chart, the astrologer can play an important role in supporting their career or some aspect of their personal development.

... AN INTELLIGENT READING OF THE BIRTH CHART CAN PAVE THE WAY FOR SELF-ACCEPTANCE AND SELF-LOVE.

How the information in the chart is delivered is fundamentally important. Certainly I have heard of cases where the information in the chart was given to the client in a deterministic way that can be crushing to the hopes and aspirations of the client coming for help. Statements such as, 'You are unlikely to ever marry' or 'You will always have problems with your health', can be very destructive and disempowering. By contrast, if the astrologer sees that there may be problems with fertility or health, he or she could impress upon the client the need to get good professional support with these issues early in the piece and may prescribe specific remedial measures to help the client overcome these possible challenges.

The astrological encounter, like any therapeutic encounter, involves two human beings and a mingling of two different energies. How these energies affect each other is often hard to predict, but is an important part of the whole equation. Importantly, as with any healthcare professional, the astrologer needs to be well trained, adept in his or her craft and have a broad experience of life. If the astrologer also has a well-developed intuition, this can further enrich the consultation.

Astrology brings its own unique way of looking at the events in a person's life. A time of isolation and aloneness may be viewed as the influence of the planet Saturn and be an important time for self-reflection, rather than cause for self-loathing and flagellation. The astrological view, while advocating a self-responsible attitude to your health and wellbeing, recognises that there are influences way beyond our personal control that play out in our lives. This can be an extremely helpful perspective, releasing the individual from the clutches of their internal critic and the tendency to take things personally. In this sense, an intelligent reading of the birth chart can pave the way for self-acceptance and self-love.

In family life, the birth chart can be a wonderful tool for understanding how our parents, partners and children are different from us. For example, why a child with strong Virgo influences in their birth chart will have an inherent need for order in their external environment so they can feel safe and secure, and why a child with a moon in Pisces will be extremely sensitive to the emotional environment in which they live. In this way, astrological information can help us in accepting, rather than judging, the individual traits of other people.

 ## The role of astrology in my life

John, a practitioner of traditional Chinese medicine and student of astrology, here shares how astrology has helped him in his career choice and in his understanding of the differing needs of his family members.

The practical use of astrology in everyday life is not what you'll get from any newspaper or magazine; however, there are a few basic concepts anyone can learn that can give valuable practical help in everyday life.

Just knowing your sun sign is enough to provide some insights. For example, in child-rearing I can see why my Capricorn (Earth sign) son loves nothing more than challenging me by arguing any theoretical point he can to prove his independence, be in control and most enjoyably for him, win the argument. Knowing this and being able to make this need of his into an intellectual game has helped diffuse what could otherwise become a very tense situation.

My Scorpio (water sign) daughter on the other hand has no interest in theoretical discussions. Her life has been led much more by her feelings. She would react to any perceived tension between family members and automatically stick up for whoever was being attacked. She needed lots of affection through physical contact whereas for the Capricorn son, there was much less need for this.

Having a Libran (air sign) wife, knowing there is a love of beauty and harmony is helpful. Our home needs to be clean and tidy for her to feel comfortable and relaxed. Also a greater need for verbal communication is needed by Librans than Capricorns, so understanding this helps to honour each other's needs.

Knowing your moon and ascendant can greatly enhance your insight into areas of your life. While studying natural therapies and exploring astrology, I found out that the placement of my sun and moon in Capricorn and rising sign in Aquarius indicated that I would be much better suited to some form of energetic healing. As acupuncture was the example given, I started to look into it and immediately felt a deep familiarity with the philosophy of Chinese medicine. By the following year I had changed colleges in order to study traditional Chinese medicine exclusively, which I have continued over the last 24 years.

Therapeutic strategies used in astrology

Astrological traditions necessarily reflect the cultures they serve. In this sense the reading you receive from a Vedic astrologer will reflect the values and culture of India, which are very different from those in the West. This may bring a whole new dimension to the reading or may seem quite irrelevant to you and the issues you are dealing with. Traditionally in India, for a woman to be told that she is likely to have difficulty in conceiving children would be unwelcome news. However, for a modern Western woman who has consciously decided not to have children, a reading of this kind may be quite in line with how she sees her life unfolding.

It is also true that Western and Vedic astrology, two astrological traditions I am familiar with, approach supporting the client in quite different ways. A remedial measure that might seem quite natural and acceptable to a person from India may seem rather peculiar to a Westerner. Where a Western astrologer may refer someone for counselling, meditation, a medical check-up or financial advice, a Vedic astrologer is more likely to prescribe specific remedies according to a time-honoured tradition.

These may include dietary recommendations, taking specific herbs, the repetition of mantras, the wearing of gemstones and the worship of planets and specific deities. Sometimes a particular pilgrimage will be prescribed, which may involve acts of charity and undertaking a sacred ritual. While some of these remedial measures may seem farfetched to someone of Western sensibility, in my experience, there is often more than a little method in the madness. For instance, committing to a specific mantra meditation practice for a period of time, when done in good faith, can go a long way to reducing anxiety and depressed mood.

The unique perspective of astrology

The beauty of an insightful reading of your birth chart is that it brings its own unique view of your personality and your life situation as it is unfolding. Your personal predicament at the time of your reading is seen as the outcome of a complex interaction between you and your environment, past and present. An interaction involving your free will as well as various cosmic forces understood through the medium of the birth chart. A skilled astrologer can assist you in understanding how these forces are currently affecting you, and how best to align yourself with these influences as you travel through life.

For example, conflict in the workplace may be seen as the result of the influence of the planet Mars transiting through the area of your chart (your tenth house) concerned with your career. Rather than blaming your workmates or berating yourself for not being able to get along with them, an astute astrologer, mindful of your chart, may be able to see which issues are being played out and how to work with them creatively. Whether you would be better served by undertaking a course in conflict resolution in order to create a more meaningful dialogue with your workmates or whether the present work environment is unlikely to suit you in the longer term.

While astrology advocates self-responsibility, it can also be tremendously helpful in not letting you take things too personally. Rather than launching into old patterns of self-recrimination and self-blame, your present difficulty is seen from a more dispassionate standpoint. This in itself can pave the way for greater self-acceptance and a more relaxed approach to life, helping you live more in the flow of life, rather than creating disasters when you are, quite literally, going 'against the stars'!

Chapter 5

Giving yourself quality time each day

Ayurveda is the knowledge that indicates the appropriate and inappropriate, happy or sorrowful conditions of living, what is auspicious or inauspicious for longevity, as well as the measure of life itself.

Charaka Samhita, textbook of Ayurvedic medicine

For many of us, travelling to exotic, faraway countries is one of life's great pleasures. Sampling the local cuisine, experiencing cultures very different from our own and taking in the sights and smells of foreign landscapes can be a most intoxicating pastime. The only downside can be dealing with the effects of jetlag when you have moved to a time zone far removed from where you normally live.

Who hasn't walked down the street of a newly arrived at city feeling like a spaced out zombie and battling the irresistible urge to sleep after a long flight? For those of us whose work involves international travel, being somewhat together for meetings in foreign countries is a further challenge. It's at times like these that a few simple measures can make an enormous difference to how you feel, your enjoyment of your holiday and how you perform if you do need to work.

Ayurveda gives us a portable toolkit of self-care practices that can be modified to suit the climate and conditions of our travel destination. Whether you are dealing with a frigid New York winter, a sweltering Mumbai before the monsoon or a misty, cool December day in Dublin, there is always something that can be done to make you feel better and more balanced.

Imagine you have just flown 20 hours from Sydney to London and after lugging your bag on and off the Heathrow Express train, have arrived at your hotel. It is 10 am on an icy, overcast February day, you did not sleep well on the flight and you just want to be horizontal and unconscious. However, you have a meeting in the afternoon and you know that you will feel groggy if you give way to sleep just now.

This is the perfect moment to bring to bear your anti-jetlag bag of tricks. First of all, drink a cup of warm water with as much awareness as you can muster. This is very pacifying to Vata dosha, which will have been aggravated by the high-speed travel on the plane, the change in climate and all the stimulation since arriving in London. Next gently stretch your body for a few minutes, reconnecting with how it feels. Then proceed to the shower recess with your plastic bottle full of sesame oil and have a hot shower. Step out of the shower stream and liberally apply some warmed oil to your whole body, making sure to spend plenty of time on the soles of your feet. When you've finished the oil massage, step back into the shower stream and let the oil wash off, leaving a thin film on your body. Towel dry, change into some loose, warm clothes and lie down on your bed. Using your smart phone and some earplugs, allow yourself to settle into a 20-minute guided meditation that encourages deep relaxation and rest.

Health tip

A hot shower and massage with sesame oil is a great way to recover your energy after a long flight.

When finished, get dressed and go about your day. If you are hungry, take a light meal that is warm and moist in its qualities. Food that is cooked and easy to digest (soup and toast is ideal) will help balance your Vata dosha and have a grounding effect. You are now much better placed to participate in your scheduled meeting and give the required presentation.

In essence, what I have described here is an approach to countering the effects of long-distance travel, which gives your body the best chance to adapt to the new time zone and environment. When these measures are embraced in a proactive manner, you are much more able to navigate through the challenges of your travel experience and be the best that you can given the circumstances. Giving yourself some quality time in this way helps keep you balanced in body and mind and enables you to enjoy, rather than suffer through, your new surrounds.

In Ayurveda, the foundation upon which health is built is known as swasthavrtta, which relates to the principles of preventive medicine. Literally translated, it means establishing yourself in healthy habits. These run through your day keeping you energetic and relaxed and preparing you for whatever the day may throw at you. They create a tone for the day and give you the best chance of meeting daily demands in a relaxed and centred way.

Essentially they are habits of self-care; caring for your body including your sense organs, your mind and your spirit. By adopting these practices, you ensure that you give yourself some 'me time' each day. Time out of your busy day to attend to your own needs, rather than the demands of your work, partner, friends or family. Allocating time each day for these practices helps your doshas stay balanced. It also allows for some kind of passive contemplation of your day and gives you time to digest the events of the day.

... ESTABLISHING A DAILY ROUTINE THAT INCLUDES SELF-CARE PRACTICES IS A SACRED DUTY.

In this sense, establishing a daily routine that includes self-care practices is a sacred duty. In caring for yourself, you are more able to impact positively with the people you share your life with, whether at work or at home. When seen in this light, these routines can be performed mindfully and can be immensely satisfying, however simple they may seem. They enable you to enter into the present moment in all its fullness, which itself is so nourishing to the spirit.

In this chapter I focus on routines for the morning and the evening, as well as routines that help prepare you for a satisfying night's sleep. The challenge is to create habits in each day and night that are enlivening, inspiring and feel good. When the routine you create for yourself is flexible and can easily be modified for the changing circumstances of your day, integrating it into your lifestyle becomes a lot easier. It is important to start where you are at, rather than set up an ambitious plan that is likely to be difficult to maintain further down the track.

In the following section I outline some of the practices recommended by Ayurveda for the morning. See which ones naturally appeal to you and consider implementing a self-care practice into your morning routine. Over time you can add to or modify your routine so that it fits in with the demands of your work and home life.

Your sacred morning routine

Ayurveda recommends waking up naturally without the use of an alarm clock, if at all possible. Once awake, rather than jumping out of bed, it suggests lying in bed for a few minutes and taking some time to connect with your body and your breath and any dreams you might have had during the night. This helps the process of embodiment and facilitates taking a more centred energy into the day ahead.

After rising from bed, it is recommended to empty your bladder, brush your teeth and gargle with water. Gandush or gargling with sesame or coconut oil for a few minutes is also advocated and helps to cleanse the mouth and nourish the gums and throat. Drinking a glass of warm water with a squeeze of lemon juice helps to pacify Vata dosha and promote a satisfying bowel habit.

Setting an intention for the day prior to undertaking some yoga stretches can be a powerful way to enter your day. Depending on how much time is available to you, these practices may take anywhere from 5 to 45 minutes, though for many people a 20-minute practice is both satisfying and do-able. Try to ensure that the yoga postures you choose are in line with your age and level of fitness. An experienced yoga teacher can help you with this and monitor your practice over time, which will need to be adjusted as you progress.

FOR MANY PEOPLE, A 20 MINUTE PRACTICE IS BOTH SATISFYING AND DOABLE.

Finishing your yoga practice with a few moments of conscious breathing or a simple yogic breathing exercise will help put you in the right space for meditation. Using whatever style of meditation you are drawn to, allow some time to sit or lie quietly. This sacred time, before the day has started, can be invaluable and helps you go into the day feeling calmer and more grounded.

After exercising, a shower or bath is recommended, depending on personal preference and time. Incorporating a quick oil massage as part of your bathing routine can be a simple and time-efficient way of nurturing yourself (see The lost art of oil self-massage on page 89). When done in the right spirit it becomes a meditation in its own right, a time to connect with your body.

Creating space so that you can have a relaxed breakfast, appropriate for the season, will also help you go into your working day feeling nourished and settled. Food entering the stomach stimulates the gastro-colic reflex, so a lot of people will feel the urge to pass a bowel motion at this point. Establishing a morning bowel habit is an important part of the natural process of detoxification each day.

Your sacred evening routine

A warm shower to wash off the accumulated energies of your working day can be a great way to transition from work to home life. Water has an innate cleansing effect and warm water helps to open up the pores of your skin and prepares you for an oil massage. Rubbing your skin with a loofah or coarse glove helps reduce any lymphatic stagnation under the skin and encourages a deeper connection with your body.

Depending on the kind of day you've had, you might like to do a few yoga stretches, especially if there is any tension in the head, neck and shoulders. This is especially common in the present age when so much time is spent on the computer and sitting for long periods. Having prepared your body in this way, some time spent in meditation or listening to a relaxing guided meditation will help clear your mind and improve your energy levels for the rest of the evening.

This is also a great time to connect with nature by watering your garden or going for a walk in your local neighbourhood, in a park or by the sea. Walking for pleasure seems to be a lost art, but walking allows you to tune into the weather, the plants and trees and the goings-on in your street, which can be immensely satisfying.

If your day has been physically active, you may prefer to sit quietly in a chair, perhaps with a cup of herbal or black tea. This simple act allows you to passively digest the day just passed and to catch up with yourself. It also can support your intuition and help you tune into its quiet voice.

Allocating time to debrief at the end of your day is time well spent. Take the time to connect with your partner, children or the people you live with and enjoy their company. The benefits of good company are extolled in Ayurvedic texts, which recognise the importance of our social needs. It is through having meaningful encounters with other people that we are reminded that we are all part of a complex web of individuals, collectively known as humanity.

Sacred routine to support a satisfying night's sleep

In the tradition of Ayurveda, once the sun goes down you are encouraged to start the process of winding down. Essentially this means avoiding, as much as possible, activities that are stimulating to the nervous system. Activities such as spending long hours on the computer, watching intense television programs or attempting to resolve conflict with your partner all increase Vata dosha and can affect the quality and quantity of your sleep. Doing more mundane and repetitive tasks around your home such as ironing, folding clothes and cleaning up the kitchen after the evening meal are advocated, and allow you to quietly digest the day just passed.

If your mind is still active going into the evening or there is something still bugging you, better to share your thoughts with your partner or ring a friend and talk things through with them. Keeping a personal journal helps get things out of your head and often brings clarity of mind. Your journal can be particularly useful when you find yourself running through an issue at 3 am. The act of putting things on paper and getting them out can help in letting the issue go and allowing you get back to sleep.

Health tip

Rubbing a little sesame oil into the soles of your feet before bedtime helps ensure a better night's sleep.

As one of my patients described to me, it will reduce the number of 'head miles' you do when lying in bed at night unable to sleep.

When there is a lot of energetic charge concentrated in the head and neck at the end of the day, getting to sleep becomes much more difficult. Gentle yoga stretches, breathing exercises and relaxation practices encourage a more even distribution of energetic charge around the body. Once this takes place and you are more connected to your body, you naturally feel any tiredness or fatigue you are carrying from the day and sleep can come quite naturally. Restorative yoga postures, such as lying face up with the length of your spine supported by a rolled up towel or bolster, can help calm the nervous system and relax the mind prior to sleep.

Foot massage, known as padabhyanga in Ayurveda, will also encourage the flow of energy away from the head and neck and into the feet. Rubbing a warmed vegetable oil such as cold-pressed sesame, almond or sunflower oil into the soles of the feet soothes the nervous system and has a deeply relaxing effect. With practice, you will find that there are certain areas on the soles of your feet that really want to be touched, so allow your intuition to guide you.

A classic Ayurvedic kitchen remedy to support a good night's sleep is to drink a cup of warm milk with a pinch of nutmeg powder added. Nutmeg has a mild sedative effect and the milk encourages blood flow into the digestive tract and away from the head. If you have an allergy to cow's milk, try goat's, soy or almond milk instead.

In Vaastu, the ancient Indian science of space harmonisation and architecture, it is said that the first image you have when you open your eyes in the morning and the last image you have when you close your eyes at night, have a strong effect on your mind. Accordingly the state of your bedroom is given considerable importance. You should feel safe and secure and enjoy its ambience. Removing the influence of technology in your bedroom, including televisions and computers, will make a significant difference to the energy of the room, as will ensuring your room is uncluttered and generally has a feeling of relaxed order. This will help to create an environment that supports a restful and nourishing night's sleep, too.

Integrating sacred routines into your life

When considering what practices you would like to include into your sacred routine, it helps when they naturally appeal to you in some way. For example, if your energy levels have been down of late, you could start by contacting a yoga teacher who you respect and ask them to put together a series of gentle stretches to be done each morning before work. Additionally you could find some relaxation music that you like, that can be played in the evenings when you get home.

Establishing your sacred routine may take some self-discipline initially, but as you begin to experience the benefits of the practices, it becomes harder not to do them. When you commit to your routine and keep it going, regardless of the dramas unfolding in your life, you begin to notice an enduring and sustaining quality present in your life. This feeling becomes stronger the more you continue to practice and refine your sacred routine.

It is important that your sacred routine fits in with the circumstances of your life. Once the principles of it are understood, your sacred routine can be adapted to the demands of shift work and night work, as in the case of individuals in occupations such as nursing and law enforcement.

In one sense, these practices encourage you to spend time with yourself – time to care for your body and mind and connect with your needs, physically, emotionally, mentally and spiritually. Many people find this difficult, but when done in the right frame of mind, these practices can profoundly transform your experience of yourself and the world around you.

In order to support your sacred routine, some people find that certain physical objects are invaluable. Useful items you might consider include:

- Aromatherapy burner
- Aromatic essential oils
- Beeswax candle
- Cards with inspirational words
- Incense sticks and holder
- Medicated massage oils
- Meditation stool or cushion
- Mementos from sacred places you have visited
- Prayer shawl
- Yoga mat or bolster.

These items can help to anchor the practice in the physical plane and their presence in your bedroom or spare room can inspire and nourish you.

For some people it will naturally feel right to create some kind of altar that can become a focus for your sacred routine. This is a very individual affair and may not appeal to some, but the presence of an altar in your living space can profoundly affect the subtle vibrations there; subtle vibrations that other people will notice when they enter your home and that support the practice of your sacred routine. As you begin to become more receptive to this dimension of experience, you will be more able to tune into the energy of people and places that you encounter in life.

My daily yoga and meditation practice

Steve, a naturopathic colleague and yoga teacher, shares his daily sacred routine, that he has carefully cultivated over many years. His approach demonstrates the principle of ahimsa, or non-violence, towards oneself and the importance of letting go of any expectations we may have about what should happen during our daily practice.

I find mornings, before breakfast, to be the best time to do my personal yoga and meditation practice. If I don't make the time in the morning, the day tends to get away from me and I have observed that I usually don't take the time during the rest of the day to do my practice.

Sometimes, I will give myself a warm oil massage using sesame seed oil medicated with herbs. This act of self-care is very special. I leave the oil on for 10 minutes or so and then shower and do my yoga practice.

I have dedicated a sacred place in a special room that is clean and spacious and which is reserved for my gentle yoga. To prepare myself, I might light some incense or a candle and perhaps read an inspirational poem, just to ease into my space.

I have a special yoga mat and a cushion to sit on and a cotton blanket to wrap myself in while I sit. Sometimes I sit on a chair.

I begin with some gentle postures that lead naturally to a breath awareness practice, which sometimes leads to a meditative state. I emphasise the word sometimes, as I don't expect a beautiful quiet, meditative state but welcome it if it arises naturally. It can occur as 'Grace' and as a natural consequence of the practice, not from my mind trying to impose itself on itself. There is no judgement around success or failure, on achieving anything. In fact in the tradition I am part of, we call it a non-achievement practice. It is done for the joy of doing it.

The immediate effect of the practice is to bring me into my body and out of my head. I am less reactive to stressful situations. I come back to my true self, hopefully without the busy monkey mind I started with. I feel grounded and nourished. The vagrant mind is reined in.

The rest of my day then seems to be gentler, calmer and easier to be in. It integrates into my life at a deeper level of self-awareness. I can be much gentler with myself, kinder to myself, and this begins to flow outwards into my life and my outer world like the ripples from a pebble thrown into a pond.

Chapter 10

The healing power of herbs

The essence of all beings is Earth. The essence of the Earth is Water. The essence of Water is plants. The essence of plants is the human being.

Chandogya Upanishad, sacred Hindu text

Low rain clouds swirled across the sky as we picked our way along the narrow path through the dense bush. Our party of four men and two boys moved steadily through the forest of low gums and paperbark trees. A light shower had fallen a few hours earlier, leaving the trees and shrubs with a fine covering of raindrops. We were en route to Bulgan, a sacred mountain to the local indigenous people, and our guide was my friend Noel Butler, a Budawang man whose family have been the traditional custodians of this land for many thousands of years.

What soon became evident as we traversed the country with Noel was that our walk that morning would also be a food gathering exercise. An opportunity to sample the local bush tucker and to nourish ourselves along the way, as many generations of his people had done before us. That morning we foraged as we walked, chewing on the stems of a local native plant that tasted a little like celery, harvesting small yellow berries from geebung trees and sucking on the exquisitely sweet nectar of moistened bottlebrush flowers; in all, an unexpected gustatory delight!

At one level we were bushwalking in fairly remote country in a national park four hours south of Sydney; at another level we were being treated to an intimate encounter with Mother Nature. Noel, through his generous sharing and his presence, was allowing us to enter into a whole different relationship with the Australian bush. A bush full of practical offerings – food, shelter and tools – and alive with spirit; not a bush to be slashed and burned but a bush to be honoured and revered as a repository of sustenance and inspiration.

In the ancient world, nature is accorded her rightful place as the giver of all life. Not something to be dominated and subjugated for the short-term gain of human beings, but something to be taken care of and protected, as you would treat your own mother. This theme of reverence and respect for the natural world is echoed in Earth-centred cultures the world over.

Near the entrance to a traditional Hindu home in India, you will find a ceramic pot containing the plant tulsi, or sacred basil. A relative of the culinary basil used worldwide, sacred basil is given a divine status and is ritually worshipped. It is known as 'the incomparable one' and is a prized medicinal herb, valued in treating lung problems, strengthening the nervous system and relieving gas in the colon. Tulsi is regarded as a consort of the god Krishna and in the ceremony of Tulsi Vivah held annually in India, Tulsi is ritually married to Krishna. By elevating tulsi in this way, the divinity in all things, including plants, is acknowledged. The fundamental place that plants occupy in the cosmic order is seen very clearly and is held to be a worthy object of worship.

> ... SACRED BASIL IS GIVEN A DIVINE STATUS AND RITUALLY WORSHIPPED.

With their astonishing ability to convert light energy into matter through the process of photosynthesis, plants enable us to draw life from the sun. They are our link to the sun and the nourishment it provides to the Earth. These facts were not lost to the ancient world which was very much aware of the primacy of the elemental world and the need to live in harmony with it. Sadly, many people in today's world have lost touch with nature.

In this chapter I look at ways in which we can cultivate a more conscious connection with the plant kingdom and all it has to offer. Plants as profound sources of nourishment – physically, emotionally, mentally and spiritually – and plants as teachers to help us regain a connection with our own essential nature.

Herbs for health and treatment

In Ayurveda, herbs are used routinely to maintain health and in the treatment of disease. Their use in healing goes back over many thousands of years and is a mainstay of contemporary Ayurvedic medical practice. Still today, my professors of Ayurvedic medicine at Gujarat Ayurveda University seek out the indigenous inhabitants of the forested areas of Gujarat to learn more about the collection and uses of various herbs.

A similar kind of interchange may also have occurred in Australia in the first few years of the penal colony established in 1788 at Port Jackson, where Sydney is now located. The native sarsparilla, a small-leafed creeper used medicinally by the local Aborigines, was the first herb exported from the colony to England. It was valued in the treatment of coughs, colds and chest complaints and the prevention of scurvy, among other things. The leaves of native sarsparilla are still used today in the form of a decoction by Aboriginal people as an aid in the treatment of diabetes.

The Ayurvedic approach to herbs is based on having an understanding of the energy of the plant. This is done through looking at the taste of the herb, how it affects the body, its effect once it has been digested by the body and knowing whether it has any special effects on certain organs of the body.

We first assess which of the six tastes (see Chapter 5) are present in a particular herb. We then look to see whether the herb has a heating or cooling effect on the body and how the effect of the herb on the body changes once it has been ingested and metabolised by the liver. Some herbs are known to have an effect on the body that cannot be explained in terms of these previous qualities, for example, turmeric is excellent for disorders of the skin – this too is taken into account. During my travels in south India, my Ayurvedic colleagues could enter a botanical garden full of herbs and simply by tasting the plant and noticing how it affected them, would then be able to suggest how it could be used medicinally.

In India, knowledge of the healing properties of herbs is not just the domain of Ayurvedic medical practitioners and village healers, it is also held in the general populace. Ask any Indian grandmother how to treat an infant's colic and she'll be quick to tell you which herb to use and how to prepare it. The women of India draw from a rich and ancient pharmacopoeia that has been passed down from mother to daughter over thousands of years. Using simple formulations of herbs and spices available in their larders and back gardens, Indian grandmothers and mothers are able to manage many common ailments in the family.

Many of these herbs and spices are freely available in the West and are routinely used in cooking. Herbs and spices such as ginger, turmeric, coriander, cinnamon and cumin have names in Sanskrit and have been used in Ayurvedic medicinal preparations for thousands of years. While a more detailed examination of medicinal kitchen herbs is beyond the scope of this book, I include a more in-depth look at turmeric and its use in healing, to give you some idea of how these kitchen herbs can be used.

Turmeric – the medicine cabinet in a jar

Turmeric, known as Haridra in Sanskrit, has been prescribed since ancient times in India and has an astonishingly wide range of medicinal uses in Ayurveda. Long prized in Indian cooking, its healing potential is now starting to be realised in Western scientific circles.

Turmeric is a tall perennial herb that grows, like ginger, from a rhizome that sits on the surface of the ground. It has a pungent and bitter taste and a warming effect on the body. It is an excellent natural antibiotic and also has antioxidant properties. It helps to strengthen the digestion and improves the quality of the bacteria in the gut.

Turmeric has a special healing power on skin diseases including acne, boils, allergic skin conditions and eczema. It promotes a healthy complexion and is an excellent blood purifier. Turmeric, with its astringent qualities, helps stop bleeding from wounds and assists in the process of healing. It is also an effective remedy for chronic cough and throat irritation.

Its anti-inflammatory action has been researched in modern times and its role in treating intestinal inflammation, ulcers, colitis and arthritis is now starting to be recognised.

It can be taken in its raw form, grated or sliced, as you would use ginger, or as a powder. If using it in its powdered form, try to get turmeric that has been recently ground, which will ensure its potency. Adding ½–1 teaspoon of turmeric powder with your other spices when cooking vegetables is a simple and effective way to bring turmeric into your diet.

Mixing a little turmeric powder with some water and making it into a paste is an excellent first aid remedy for itchy skin conditions – just gently rub the paste into the affected area of skin. I have even found it extremely useful in relieving the persistent itch that comes after a leech bite!

I include below an Ayurvedic herbal tea that is a good way to include turmeric into your diet, especially in winter. It is spicy and warming, has a cleansing effect on the body, stimulates the digestion and is useful in treating coughs and colds.

2–3 slices fresh turmeric
1 teaspoon fenugreek seeds
1 teaspoon cloves (omit if Pitta-dominant body type)
1 teaspoon dill seeds

◎ Put all the ingredients in a teapot, add 3–4 cups of boiling water and let steep for 3 minutes.
◎ Please note that if symptoms persist in spite of treatment, it is important to see your trusted local health practitioner for further assessment and advice.

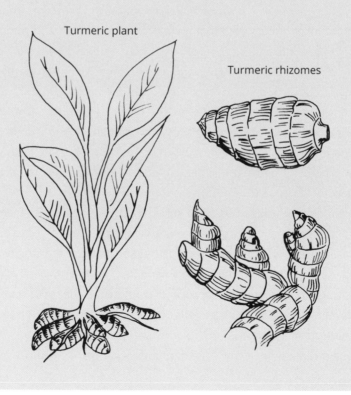

Turmeric plant

Turmeric rhizomes

Kitchen herbs and the digestive fire

In Chapter 5 I discussed the close link between the agni, or digestive fire, and immune-system functioning. In Ayurveda kitchen herbs and spices are one way of strengthening a low or irregular digestive fire or balancing an excessively strong digestive fire.

Generally individuals with a predominant Vata body type are prone to irregular digestion and irregular bowel movements. If their Vata dosha becomes aggravated, they may experience constipation, excessive wind, bloating and abdominal distension. Their digestion fire can easily be overwhelmed and can be regularised by adding herbs and spices to their diet. Herbs and spices such as cumin, mustard seed, coriander, turmeric, ginger and curry leaf are recommended, though very heating spices such as chilli, clove and too much black pepper can create dryness in the colon and constipation.

Individuals with a predominant Pitta body type have a strong digestion. If their Pitta dosha becomes aggravated, they may experience heartburn, hyper-acidity and ulceration in the gut. Their digestive fire can create inflammation of the lining of the gut and needs to be balanced with cooling spices. Herbs and spices such as coriander, fennel, gotu cola and liquorice root are recommended. Small amounts of turmeric, ginger and cumin are also beneficial. Western herbs such as oregano, basil, parsley and mint are ideal for Pitta body types.

> KITCHEN HERBS AND SPICES ARE ONE WAY OF STRENGTHENING A LOW OR IRREGULAR DIGESTIVE FIRE ...

Individuals with a predominant Kapha body type have a low digestive fire. If their Kapha dosha becomes aggravated, they may experience mucus build-up in the body, fluid retention and the accumulation of fat. Their digestive fire responds to all herbs and spices but particularly to hot and stimulating ones, including chilli, clove and black pepper.

It is important to check out how you are feeling before selecting the herbs and spices to be used in your cooking. In this way you can fine-tune which feel right for you at a particular time. This makes for a more flexible approach and allows room for your intuition to have its say.

Some common kitchen herbs and their use in healing in Ayurveda

I include here a list of kitchen herbs and spices that are used in Ayurveda to balance the digestion and promote wellbeing. Each herb has a number of specific properties that can be helpful in treating minor health imbalances. For example, ginger is very helpful in the treatment of nausea and has been safely used by pregnant mothers with morning sickness for thousands of years. By using them mindfully in your cooking, kitchen herbs and spices can play an important role in preventive medicine.

For each herb, I first include the name in English and then the Sanskrit name in brackets. The predominant taste or tastes are then given, followed by its effect on the body, in terms of whether it is heating or cooling. I then give a brief account of its specific medicinal qualities.

Asafoetida (hingu) is pungent in taste and has a heating effect on the body. It is a resinous gum that comes from a giant fennel plant grown in Kashmir and Afghanistan. It warms the digestive tract and promotes assimilation of nutrients and circulation. When using it in your cooking, add a pinch of asafoetida powder to hot oil before adding whole seeds such as cumin and mustard for frying. It is used as a substitute for onion and garlic in some Hindu spiritual traditions. Cooking with asafoetida makes legumes more digestible. A word of caution: it should not be used in pregnancy or when Pitta is aggravated in the body.

Black pepper (maricha) is pungent in taste and has a heating effect on the body. It stimulates the agni and has a detoxifying effect on the body. It is useful in sinus congestion and when Kapha dosha is aggravated in the body. It is an antioxidant.

Cardamom (ela) is pungent and sweet in taste and has a slightly warming effect on the body. It is an excellent digestive and is useful for reducing mucus in the body and in the treatment of nausea. It helps repair the lining of the lungs.

Cinnamon (twak) is pungent, sweet and astringent in taste. It has a warming effect on the body. It increases vitality, calms the digestive process, aids peripheral circulation and is useful in menstrual and abdominal cramps.

Coriander (dhanyaka) is bitter and pungent in taste and has a cooling effect on the body. It is useful in strengthening the digestion, helps to stabilise the blood sugar, and is useful in the relief of urinary tract infections. Coriander leaf juice is also useful in treating allergy.

Cumin (jiraka) is pungent and bitter in taste and has a cooling effect on the body. It is a useful anti-gas remedy and helps stimulate the digestion. Cumin water is used in hot weather to stay cool. As a drink, it is also helpful in the treatment of haemorrhoids.

Fennel (sampf) is sweet and pungent in taste and has a cooling effect on the body. Fennel has a soothing effect on digestive upset caused by gas and irritation in the bowel. It promotes lactation and stabilises the blood sugar level in the body. In India lactating mothers drink fennel tea to help prevent colic in babies.

Fenugreek (methi) is bitter, pungent, sweet in taste and has a heating effect on the body. An excellent digestive, it helps settle gas and inflammation in the gut. Useful in the treatment of sore throats, sinusitis and is said to help in lowering cholesterol levels.

Garlic (lasunam) possesses all six tastes but sour and has a heating effect on the body. It is anti-bacterial, anti-parasitic and is used to treat ear infections, stimulate the immune system, detoxify the body, increase stamina, reduce mucus and increase the libido. It helps to pacify Vata dosha and support the immune system.

Ginger (ardraka – fresh) is pungent and sweet in taste and has a heating effect on the body. It is called the universal medicine in Ayurveda and has many uses. It stimulates the agni, increases circulation, reduces mucus in the lungs, and helps in the treatment of nausea. It is widely used in the treatment of arthritis and in promoting healthy metabolism of fats in the body.

Mustard (rajika) is pungent in taste and has a heating effect on the body. A warming carminative, it helps settle digestive upset and is useful in the treatment of coughs and in reducing mucus in the body. Brown mustard is less heating than yellow mustard.

Nutmeg (jatiphala) is pungent in taste and has a heating effect on the body. It is a useful digestive, especially in the treatment of diarrhoea (administer a quarter of a teaspoon in a cup of buttermilk) and enhances the circulation. Nutmeg is useful in the treatment of insomnia (a pinch in a cup of warm milk before bed), having a sedating effect. It has aphrodisiac properties.

Saffron (kesar) is pungent, bitter and sweet in taste and has a cooling effect on the body. It has been used for over 3600 years for a variety of conditions. It is a potent blood revitaliser and enhances the circulation. It is used in treatment of disorders of the female reproductive system including infertility and menstrual problems.

Herbal teas to balance Vata, Pitta and Kapha dosha

Teas are another easy way to introduce herbs into your diet. I recommend using a coffee plunger and flask and adding the fresh or dried herbs and boiling water to it. The herbal teas below are just a starting point for your own experimentation. Find out which kitchen herbs and spices make you feel good and try a few different variations.

To get the maximum benefit from these infusions it is best to be sitting down when drinking them, to sip mindfully and notice how the tea affects you physically, emotionally and mentally. The recipes below are for a coffee flask or teapot catering for four to five people.

Vata balancing tea

2 cm fresh ginger, peeled and sliced
1 cinnamon quill
1 teaspoon dried liquorice root pieces
    or fennel seeds

Pitta balancing tea

1 teaspoon fennel seeds
1 teaspoon coriander seeds
5–6 cardamom pods
2 sprigs fresh mint leaves

Kapha balancing tea

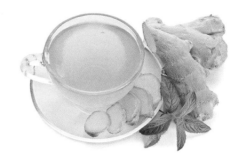

2 cm fresh ginger, peeled and sliced
1 teaspoon fenugreek seeds
½ teaspoon cloves
¼ teaspoon turmeric powder
¼ teaspoon peppercorns

Cultivating your home herb and vegetable garden

Creating and managing your own herb and/or vegetable garden is another way to allow the plant kingdom to enter your life. As all gardeners know, watching plants grow and tending to their needs is an extraordinarily satisfying endeavour and brings a more sensitive understanding of the natural world. It gives a firsthand and intimate opportunity to see how Mother Nature works and ties us into the cycles of the day and night, the weather, the seasons and the cycle of the moon.

The needs of plants are relatively simple: the right type of soil, adequate water, suitable temperature and the right amount of sun go a long way to helping them grow and thrive. Ensuring that the right conditions are met for a particular plant requires a little knowledge and the regular observation of the plant and how it is faring. Establishing a home composting bin using leftover vegetable and fruit scraps, grass cuttings and leaves will help you create a nourishing soil for your herbs and vegetables. It also means that less organic matter is going into plastic bags that will end up in landfill sites on the outskirts of the city you live in.

Time spent outdoors weeding and watering your herbs and vegetables helps you to connect with your local environment and meet your neighbours. Gardening helps you to ground your energy and connect with the earth and as such is a natural antidote to the hours spent interacting with computer screens and other technological devices.

Even apartment dwellers can cultivate their own herb garden on a windowsill or balcony and use home-grown herbs to enliven their meals. It is amazing to me how much better a pasta sauce or salad tastes when you add your own parsley, basil or chives to the mix. Participating in a community garden adds a whole other dimension to the gardening experience, bringing you into contact with like-minded people and enabling you to benefit from fresh, organically grown ingredients.

At one point in my career, I was involved with a community garden run a stone's throw from the University of New South Wales in Sydney. The garden occupied a large suburban block and was tended by volunteer students of botany and biology from the university. It utilised the grey water from the washing machine and kitchen sink of an adjoining house, and horse manure and hay from nearby Randwick racecourse. The garden also ran chickens whose droppings also helped fertilise the soil. Drawing from the principles of permaculture, the garden grew a wide variety of plants including fruit trees, vegetables and legumes. It was managed by a young man with a passion for sustainable living and is a wonderful example of what is possible when vision and collective will are combined.

 ## Healing in your back garden

Jennifer, an Ayurvedic colleague of mine, has embraced healing using herbs grown in the garden of her suburban home. Jennifer's small front garden is a meadow of a diverse range of herbs that she uses to an extraordinary degree to support her own healthcare needs and those of her family, including Winnie her 13-year-old Labrador.

What we classify as weeds have been used from the days of the caveman to present times; herbs have been used to promote and safeguard health and to heal disease in people as well as our domesticated animals.

I set out to cultivate a garden of herbs, vegetables and flowers that attracted bird life, butterflies, ladybirds and bees. And I stopped pruning my garden of weeds such as dandelion, nettle, comfrey, violet, plantain and chickweed and let them grow wild in the garden.

Dandelion is a wonderful herb for blood, lymph and liver. Dandelion cools and clears the liver of congestion. After a few weeks of eating dandelion, many commented that I had lost weight. I realised the dandelion had removed all my bloated, distended midriff, which is so common in middle-aged woman. What an easy way to lose weight and keep it off!

Add dandelion to a salad or use as a garnish. Dandelion leaf infused in a glass of wine for one hour prior to drinking protects the liver from the effects of alcohol, softens the acidic taste of the wine and aids digestion.

Stinging nettle nourishes the adrenals. Within a few days of consuming stinging nettle in dry infusions, rice, dahl and vegetable dishes, I felt a boost of energy and needed less sleep. I felt calm. My hair, skin and nails where glowing, thicker and stronger. Even my golden Labrador Winnie had a glowing soft coat after having her coat rinsed with nettle infusion. Nettle also increased my libido.

I had some arthritis in my right hip and scoliosis in the spine. Winnie had arthritis in her hind legs, finding it difficult to climb up stairs. So we both started to have dried comfrey infusions and I added comfrey as a green to all dishes that were suitable. We both experienced relief from our aches and pains.

Violet leaves are superb nourishment, supporting the liver, gall bladder, digestive and urinary system. Violet's expectorant effects are very useful for coughs, congestion and inflamed throats when used as a tea and poultice to the affected area. Very useful for monthly sore/ tender breasts prior to menstruation as well. I use violet leaves fresh in salads and tea.

Plantain gives speedy relief when applied to all kinds of bites and stings, and is good for all skin ailments; apply the crushed leaves directly to skin/wounds. I came in from the garden one day with a rash all over the top of my right hand. I applied crushed plantain leaf with some saliva and covered it with a crepe bandage, and within a few hours the rash was gone.

Chickweed is another weed I would always pull from the garden, but it's fantastic fresh in a salad or just eaten raw from the garden. Chickweed is an old wives' remedy for obesity as it is said to dissolve fat. It is a superb metabolic balancer and has a regulating effect on the thyroid. Chickweed is also a joint oiler, and hot chickweed baths, soaks and poultices relieve sore back, legs, gout, backache and bursitis.

What I have experienced by living and being in the garden is that optimal nourishment is whole, holy, vital, wild, unique, local, common, simple, messy, fresh, abundant, accessible, seasonal, varied and full of love.

Our attitude to nature

Ayurveda advocates living in harmony with nature. By nature, it refers not just to the external world of plants, animals, landforms and the weather, but also our own nature. We too are part of nature and are encouraged to develop a relationship with ourselves that is harmonious. A relationship where we honour our own needs as individuals, while not forgetting that we are part of an intricate web of relationship with both animate and inanimate objects.

Nature is viewed as a much-cherished friend. As such it is prudent to listen to her and the messages she is giving us from moment to moment, messages about the state of the natural world as well as messages from our own bodies.

By contrast, the attitude to nature that has developed in post-industrial, technology-driven societies, where consumerism is the order of the day, is based on dominating nature. Nature is viewed as a resource to be exploited in the service of the short-term needs of man. Seen in this light, her needs are not understood, not valued and are deemed to be of secondary importance. While it is true that scientific research is beginning to plumb the depths of her complexity, too often short-term political agendas and the needs of multinational corporations requiring profits for shareholders hold sway.

This way of relating to nature is, not surprisingly, reflected in how we relate to our bodies. As individuals, we learn at an early age to suppress and override our natural bodily reactions and emotional responses to situations. We have lost touch with ourselves and this becomes an habitual way of being. It's a way of being that involves a fundamental level of disconnection, a disconnection from our bodies and from the natural world that has sustained us for so long.

As a result, our capacity to think and act wisely as a species has become impoverished. At a time when a caring and careful approach to nature is most needed, we are no longer sensitive and responsive to her cries for help.

The experience of managing a herb and/or vegetable garden throughout the year allows for a more intimate encounter with the plant world and nature in general. In my own case, it has led to encounters with fruit bats, possums and a blue-tongue lizard and an appreciation of an array of birds that frequent the part of Sydney I live in, including rainbow lorikeets, magpies, kookaburras, crows and minors. I now know that the yellow-tailed black cockatoo, with its haunting, primeval cry, comes to our suburb from April through to October in search of banksias and other plant food. A natural consequence of these experiences is a greater awareness of how our society interacts with nature and the extent to which a lot of our societal structures show a fundamental lack of respect for her welfare.

The stark contrast in attitude between ancient and modern cultures to the natural world was highlighted for me during a visit to a pristine mountain rainforest in Dorrigo National Park in New South Wales. The local Gumbaynggirr Aborigines described the canopy of the rainforest as 'a blanket over the land that protects the earth', whereas for the first Europeans, the forest was simply 'thick impenetrable scrub'.

The fact that Australia's indigenous peoples have been largely excluded from the process of deciding how best to manage our national parks, and our relationship with nature in general in this country is astounding and evidence of how little things have changed over the past two centuries. The accumulated wisdom of 70,000 years of continued habitation of this land could only enrich the process of making policies that ensure that country is safeguarded for future generations of Australians.

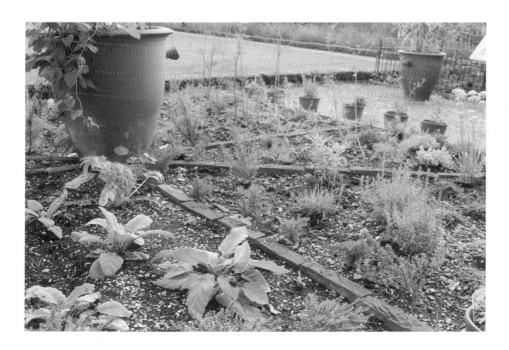

chapter II

The secrets of eternal youth

Rasayana [the science of rejuvenation] is possessed of inconceivable and wonderful possibilities, being promotive of longevity and health, preservation of youth, and ridding the body of sleepiness, fatigue, exhaustion and weakness.

Ashtanga Hridayam, Ayurvedic medical text

It was mid-morning on a weekday and I had come to the aged-care facility to visit a close family relative suffering from Alzheimer's disease. I had arrived at the special care unit, a locked ward catering to the needs of patients with moderately severe dementia, to find that my relative was not quite ready to leave the ward with me for our customary drive and coffee. While she was being attended to by the nursing staff, I found a chair in the corner of the recreational area of the unit and waited quietly.

There were a few other patients in the open plan room, most of whom were asleep in their chairs, though there was one elderly woman who was quite agitated. I had observed her on previous visits to the ward, sometimes making unintelligible repetitive sounds for hours on end and often seeming to be in a state of considerable distress. I had never seen her being able to verbally communicate and despite the attentions of the staff, very little seemed to relieve her obvious suffering. It was very difficult to watch and at times, her plight would just be in the background of the daily routines and goings on in the ward.

This day, however, I sat and watched as one of the nursing staff, a Nepali man who had recently immigrated to Australia with his wife and young family, came over and began to gently massage her head. He did this quite naturally and she immediately responded to his touch and the contact he was offering. Soon her whole demeanour changed and her face was beaming with obvious enjoyment. Sitting there that morning, I was deeply moved by his compassionate act and the seemingly effortless and tender way in which he attended to her needs.

In this particular facility, many of the nursing staff come from countries such as India, Nepal, the Phillipines, China and Fiji. Countries where the traditional culture honours its old people and places a high value on the care of the elderly. In retrospect, it was no accident that this particular man was very comfortable giving his patient a head massage given that Ayurveda runs through the fabric of society in the Nepal. Indeed the word shampoo in English is derived from the Hindi word champi, which means head massage, and is a therapeutic practice employed by masseurs and even barbers across the length and breadth of the Indian sub-continent.

In this chapter I explore how Ayurveda understands the phenomenon of ageing and how we can rejuvenate our bodies and minds by making changes to our diet and lifestyle, and embracing therapies that slow down the ageing process.

> IN AYURVEDA, THE FIRST 30 YEARS OF OUR LIFE IS HELD TO BE UNDER THE INFLUENCE OF KAPHA DOSHA.

In Ayurveda, the first 30 years of our life is held to be under the influence of Kapha dosha. This is when we are at our most juicy, our skin is soft and well hydrated, our body more rounded with puppy fat and we are more prone to mucus in the form of coughs and colds. The next 30 years are held to be under the influence of Pitta dosha. This is when we are most productive and dynamic and when our bodies heat up. It is the time of menopause in women with the associated symptoms of intolerance to heat and hot flushes. After the age of 60, Vata dosha is the dominant dosha in our lives. Under its influence, we begin to dry up, both internally and externally. This process affects the whole body, resulting in conditions such as dry skin, stiff joints, brittle bones, poor memory, reduced hearing, eyesight and weakened internal organs.

Ayurveda comprises eight limbs, one of which is known as Rasayana – the art and science of rejuvenation. Rasayana, translated literally, means 'the path of juice'. It concerns itself with how to best nourish our bodily fluids and in simple terms how to make ourselves more juicy. Rasayana self-care practices and treatments aim to counterbalance the drying effects of Vata dosa and thereby slow down the ageing process, and improve both the quality and length of our lives.

Moderation in all things

During my travels in India I met with a number of individuals who were living their lives in line with many of the principles in this book. They tended to come from families where Ayurveda and yoga had been embraced for many generations and this had resulted in a way of being that produced very little wear and tear on the body and mind. It was not uncommon for me to encounter people who looked like they were in their sixties, but in fact were well into their ninth decade of life.

I also had the opportunity to stay in their homes and observe first-hand their diet and lifestyle and how they lived as families. What soon became obvious to me was how they were acutely aware of the effect of food on their overall health, in terms of both the quality and quantity of what they were consuming. A great deal of attention went into the preparation of food and the sharing of food was always an occasion of importance in their daily lives.

They neither drank nor smoked and had an established morning routine that often involved some form of gentle stretching or breathing exercises and a period of meditation or study of sacred texts. In India, where the elderly tend to be revered and have an integral role in family life, it is the custom to live with your extended family. It is quite common for grandparents to be looking after young children at home while their parents are off at work.

Each extended family would have strong contacts with maternal and paternal relatives who they would visit from time to time. The extended family would also go on holiday together; invariably this would entail a pilgrimage to a sacred place or temple in another part of India. This would allow for quality family time together, removed from the humdrum of daily life.

In all, I was struck by the strength of the social fabric that underpinned the lives of these people; lives that were being lived with a degree of moderation and balance that I do not often encounter in the West. I came away with the feeling that the lifestyles they were living were nourishing on many levels, contributing in large part to the quality of life they were enjoying. It was also apparent that we in the West could learn much from their habits and practices, given our ageing population and the costs of looking after their healthcare needs.

Rejuvenation through self-care practices

In many ways Ayurveda is a handbook of self-care practices that encourage us to stay more connected to our essential nature. One that is innately healing and peaceful. Ayurveda also recognises the need to use its principles in ways that are appropriate for the society in which it is being practised and the age. As such there are many practices that are innately rejuvenating in their effect and which can be incorporated into a modern lifestyle. Here I look at some of these practices in greater detail.

Meditation practices, through their ability to quieten the monkey mind and bring us to a place of stillness, are foremost among rejuvenation practices. While finding the practice that really speaks to you and allows you to connect with the timeless present is a highly individual affair, I do find that lying down meditation practices that focus on the body are particularly useful. Even sitting up requires a degree of energy expenditure whereas a lying down meditation allows for a deeper level of relaxation. The nervous system can rest and the digestion can settle more easily when you are lying on your back.

Health tip

A regular and satisfying practice of meditation is one of the most powerful ways to rejuvenate body and mind.

Naturally it is important that you feel safe and secure in the place where you are meditating. In practical terms, this means making sure you won't be interrupted during your practice and that you are comfortable with the energy of the room. It then becomes more possible, especially in the early stages of your practice, to completely surrender to the experience of meditation.

In our busy modern lives, many people are running on adrenaline and suffering from chronic depletion. The running-on-empty feeling is endemic and only aggravated by the consumption of stimulants such as tea and coffee. In my experience very few people know how to truly rest. By rest I mean being able to relax the whole body, including the organs in the abdomen. Stress is not just held in the muscles and joints of the body but in the organs of digestion, as discussed in the chapter on the digestive fire. Learning how to relax these deeper levels of tension in the body is not something that is taught in school and requires specific training – training from someone well versed in the technique and who has been using the practice in their daily life for some time.

As discussed in Chapter 6, it is important to prepare the body prior to the practice of meditation. This is where body–mind integration practices such as yoga postures, tai chi, yogic breathing practices and qigong are invaluable in releasing stress, energising the body and quietening the mind.

(IN MY EXPERIENCE VERY FEW PEOPLE KNOW HOW TO TRULY REST.)

Self-oil massage can also be very useful in this regard and can be incorporated in your shower routine. The combination of a hot shower, self-massage with oil and listening to a relaxing meditation is a great way to transition from your work day to time at home with your partner, family or flatmates.

In Ayurveda, the first line of treatment is to remove the cause of the condition, so in order to rejuvenate we must also be mindful of those behaviours that cause us to leak vital energy or prana. Recreational drug use, burning the candle at both ends, late nights, excessive sexual activity, and long hours on the computer or at work will all aggravate Vata dosha and accelerate the ageing process.

In essence rejuvenation is very much about how you manage your energy from moment to moment. Are you living a lifestyle that is depleting your energy levels or one where you are consciously conserving your energy? Self-care practices remind you to connect with your bodily needs and encourage you to nurture yourself as you proceed through life. In this sense rejuvenation is firmly based in the principles of preventive medicine rather than a toolbox for rectifying worn-out parts. I include a list of self-care practices that have been found useful by many of my patients, students and colleagues over the years.

Some additional practical approaches to rejuvenation

Drinking a cup of herbal tea mindfully

Completing tasks

Getting to bed early

Saying 'no'

Avoiding multi-tasking

Being present

Sex in moderation

Regular holidays/retreats

Music that sustains you

Slowing down

Turning your phone off

Having a relaxing bath with oils/salts

Hobbies

Contact with nature

Gardening

Conversations with friends

Quality time with partner, family or friends

 ## Managing body–mind for Vatas

Philippa, a 62-year old mother of four who works as a library assistant, shares her experience of having a Vata dominant body type and how she understands and manages her body–mind health in ways that keep her balanced through her day.

Vata is a more predominant dosha for me. Now that I have an understanding of Ayurvedic philosophy I realise that the way in which I have reacted to situations and experiences throughout my life – and also a number of issues I have had with my physical body – are a result of having a predominant Vata dosha or one that has been aggravated and is then out of balance.

One area where I am conscious of the way Vata or excess Vata energy can be felt in the body is in the mind and around mental processing. Having a mind that is often very active and at various times overactive I can be prone to overthinking situations, which can then lead to states of worry, anxiety and feelings of insecurity.

My sleeping routine is typical of Vata or aggravated Vata. While I usually go to sleep quite quickly I often sleep very lightly and am prone to waking during the night and having difficulty going back to sleep. Frequently the waking will be accompanied by thoughts of a topic that is currently on my mind. I also find excessive wind for long periods, loud noise, highly populated places or those congested by people or traffic to be quite aggravating, leaving me feeling more tense, disconnected and spacey.

Another area of the body that is ruled by Vata is pain, especially in the joints. I suffered from this since I was six years old, fortunately without swelling or disfiguration. As a child it was confined to my knees but after my mother's illness and death in my late teenage years, a time of considerable trauma, it spread to many joints throughout my body. I have been able to see how episodes of increased pain have been connected to periods of increased stress and anxiety, and increased Vata activity. I have also noticed how remissions are related to calmer and more balanced times in my life.

During our life journey we are exposed to and experience many situations that challenge us emotionally but this is how we learn valuable lessons. We cannot prevent this from happening but we can adopt practices that will help us to manage when these situations occur and when our doshas are thrown out of balance as a result. Having an understanding of Ayurvedic practices has allowed me to recognise when there is imbalance and has given me tools to address this.

To help counteract the air energy of my Vata dosha I make sure I include root vegetables in my diet and choose these and cooked vegetables in general in preference to lighter and uncooked ones. To help with the drying effects I am conscious of consuming adequate fluids, especially water. I have in the past been prone to eating too quickly and not always sitting down to eat. By having more awareness of the importance of eating more slowly and calmly I have experienced less digestive disturbances. If possible, I also minimise exposure to noise and crowds. This can be as simple as choosing to eat out at restaurants that are quieter or to eat on less busy nights of the week.

I also find a regular meditation practice and regular massages a great benefit. These two practices in particular I find helpful in aiding my sleep routine. While I am attracted to more active and vigorous forms of exercise, during times when I feel that this dosha is aggravated, I try to choose more grounding ways of exercising such as Pilates or yoga. If I feel agitated or anxious I try to stay away from activities that will fuel these feelings.

Understanding why I react or feel the way I do at different times and then adopting the appropriate practices of Ayurveda helps me to balance my emotions and mind and ultimately my physical body.

Health maintenance – being proactive in rejuvenating your mind and body

Many years ago I found myself having Christmas at an Ayurvedic retreat centre in south India. The centre was set in the midst of rural India and had residential treatment facilities for about fifteen patients. Some of the people there were suffering from chronic illnesses such as rheumatoid arthritis and stroke-induced paralysis, but others were there for health maintenance.

One Indian couple I met, who were both in their late sixties and in reasonable health, came to the retreat centre for two weeks every year to rejuvenate. He had mild maturity onset diabetes and she had mild hypertension. While staying at the treatment facility they would be put on a simple whole food diet, be prescribed Ayurvedic herbal treatments and receive daily warm oil massage treatments that encourage both detoxification and rejuvenation. This had been their practice for several years and enabled them to have plenty of time to write letters, catch up on some reading and relax. The retreat centre was situated in the midst of rice paddies, coconut groves and patches of tropical forest, so there was also opportunity for relaxing walks in nature and time for passive contemplation.

As well as practising moderation in their daily diet and lifestyle, they recognised the need to devote time out of their busy family lives to support their physical, emotional and mental wellbeing. Using these approaches, they were both able to successfully manage their illnesses and prevent any further complications from developing.

My experience as a holistic general practitioner and Ayurvedic therapist practising in the West is quite different. Often I see patients with chronic illnesses who are relying heavily on medication to treat their degenerative disease process and have not embraced the need for dietary, lifestyle and attitudinal change in their lives. 'Same old, same old' rules the day, until they reach a point where additional medical intervention is required in order to control their symptoms, intervention that may involve surgery or stronger medication with unpleasant side effects. The doctor is seen as someone who can fix your health problems rather than the patient taking responsibility for their own health and wellbeing.

This situation, to some extent, does reflect the training of medical practitioners in Western medicine where the major focus is on the treatment of disease. Traditionally, little time in the curriculum of medical school was devoted to preventive medicine and no time was devoted to wellbeing. By contrast Ayurveda, with its broad scope, has developed time-tested and sophisticated approaches to the promotion of wellbeing. Fortunately many medical schools are now embracing the bio–psycho–social model of health, which looks at health in much broader terms. In this model the doctor is actively involved in enabling the patient through education in healthy diet and lifestyle practices.

The five deep-cleansing practices of Ayurveda

Just as a cloth is cleaned of any impurities prior to dying it another colour, so some level of detoxification is advocated prior to the process of rejuvenation. This is particularly so when undergoing more intensive rejuvenating processes, which are usually done in a residential setting such as an Ayurvedic health retreat. The process begins with a detailed health and lifestyle assessment by an Ayurvedic physician. During the treatment program, which could take from one week to several months depending on the condition being treated, you are assessed each day by the physician, so that the program can be adjusted as necessary to best suit your needs.

Ayurveda has devised five deep-cleansing practices known as Panchakarma to facilitate purification of the body and mind and to prepare both for rejuvenation. There are three stages to this detoxifying process.

First the body is oleated or saturated with oil using daily warm oil massage and through drinking ghee (clarified butter), which serves to soften aggravated doshas in the tissues. The body is then made to sweat through the use of steam boxes and sweating therapies, which help the aggravated doshas to melt. This enables the disease-producing or 'morbid' doshas to enter the blood stream and return to their home in the body. In the case of Vata, these morbid doshas are brought to the large bowel, while in Pitta these morbid doshas are brought to the small intestine, and in the case of Kapha they are brought to the stomach.

Once this has been achieved, a process that may take several days to a week, the five deep-cleansing practices can be performed. In general terms, when Kapha dosha has become aggravated emesis therapy, which involves induced vomiting, is prescribed; when Pitta dosha has become aggravated purgation is prescribed; and when Vata dosha has become aggravated, herbal decoction and oily enema are prescribed. Specific Ayurvedic herbs are utilised to induce vomiting, purgation and in the enemas. Using these techniques the disease-producing doshas are expelled from the body, allowing for a profound level of detoxification and purification.

During the process of oleation and sweating therapies patients are put on a light diet along with Ayurvedic medicinal herbs and are encouraged to take every opportunity to rest. On the day of the emesis or purgation therapies, the patient would be fasting and the next day would take only rice gruel and warm water.

The last deep-cleansing practice in Panchakarma is known as nasya karma (nasal therapies). Nasya karma involves the application of medicated oil drops to the nasal passages, after preliminary treatment to the head and neck with oil massage and hot compresses. It is particularly useful in the treatment of head and neck diseases including headaches and migraines.

The final stage of these deep-cleansing therapies involves following a diet appropriate for your body type, ongoing herbal treatment and plenty of rest.

What I have described here are therapeutic processes that should only be undertaken when under the care of an Ayurvedic physician with plenty of experience in these therapies and in a centre that is fully equipped to deal with the likely needs of the patient. The five deep-cleansing therapies are an important arm of Ayurvedic therapeutics, both in the treatment of chronic disease and as a prelude to rejuvenating therapies in healthy people.

NASYA KARMA IS PARTICULARLY USEFUL IN THE TREATMENT OF HEAD AND NECK DISEASES INCLUDING HEADACHES AND MIGRAINES.

A previous student of mine witnessed the power of Panchakarma while receiving treatment at an Ayurvedic clinic in Mumbai. One of her fellow patients was a concert pianist who had been struck down with rheumatoid arthritis, a potentially crippling disease that had affected her hands severely. On the final day of her three-month treatment program, the young woman played an entire piano concerto for the assembled staff and patients at the clinic.

Rejuvenation using oil massage

Once Panchakarma is completed, further rejuvenating oil massage treatments are prescribed. Massage, whether received or given to yourself, is an important aspect of the practice of rejuvenation in Ayurveda. Touch is an important way to convey vital energy or prana. So both self-massage and receiving a massage helps revitalise not just the physical body but also the mind and the heart. The application of the oil, given the absorptive quality of our skin, also has the effect of oleating the inner environment of our body.

In Ayurveda, oil massage is known as abhyanga. In abhyanga, 300 ml of warm, herbally medicated oils are applied to the body on a specially designed table known as a droni. The warm oil is massaged into the body over a period of 45 minutes by one or two massage therapists. The oil and the herbs contained in it are absorbed through the skin and enter the circulation of the body. During the massage specific marma or vital energy points, similar to acupressure points in traditional Chinese medicine, are also stimulated. Thus these massage practices act at the physical as well as the subtle level to nourish depleted tissues and organs and to restore balance in the body. In this way external massage has a direct healing effect on the internal organs and the flow of prana in the body. The cumulative effect of the massage treatment is to counteract dryness in the body and slow down the ageing process.

In recent years, a powerful rejuvenating treatment known as shirodhara has become popular in the West. In shirodhara, 2 litres of warm oil is poured in a gentle, steady stream across the forehead and scalp over a period of 45 minutes from a vessel held several centimetres above the patient's head. This has a profoundly relaxing effect on the nervous system. Once you get used to the procedure, its effect can last for days and even weeks. When given on a daily basis for 7, 14 or 21 days it produces long-lasting shifts in the physiology of the body. Shirodhara is used in Ayurveda to treat generalised stress, anxiety, insomnia and high blood pressure.

There are a number of other massage practices used to rejuvenate the tissues of the body. In pizichile, 2 litres of warm medicated oil, appropriate for your body type and any underlying health conditions, is massaged into the body by two massage therapists working in synchrony. This treatment is profoundly oleating to the body and initially produces a feeling of heaviness. In order to receive the full benefit from pizichile, it is important to take plenty of time after the treatment to rest and sleep as necessary. The treatment is best undertaken while staying in a residential facility such as an Ayurvedic health retreat.

Nawarakidhi, also known as rice pudding massage, is another deeply nourishing treatment used in Ayurveda. A pudding made from a certain kind of rice, milk and a nourishing herb is cooked up and put into small pouches of muslin. These pouches are then dipped in warm milk and used to massage the body using a combination of long flowing strokes and small circular movements. Nawarakidhi has a cooling effect on the body and is useful when there is excess heat in the body. It's also beneficial when the body's organs have become depleted and for the treatment of certain kinds of paralysis.

Ayurvedic massage oils

Specific massage oils are selected in Ayurveda, depending on the inherent qualities of the oil and whether it will suit the client. In this regard, the constitution of the client, the state of their general health and the season in which the massage is being given will be taken into consideration. In general terms, individuals with a Vata-dominant constitution tend to do best with warming, heavier oils such as sesame or almond oil; those with a Pitta-dominant constitution tend to do best with cooling oils such as sunflower or coconut oil; and those with a Kapha-dominant constitution tend to do best with a light, warming oil such as safflower oil.

In order to enhance the therapeutic effect of oil massage, Ayurveda also makes use of massage oils medicated with specific herbs. Base oils such as sesame or coconut are medicated using decoctions of various herbs so that the properties of the herbs enter into the oils, enhancing their therapeutic effect. Many of the herbs used are tonics that are particularly nourishing to the body such as ashwagandha (*Withania somnifera*) and shatavari (*Asparagus racemosus*). Other herbs are specifically nourishing to the nervous system, such as gotu cola (*Centella asiatica*) and brahmi (*Bacopa monniera*).

A number of these herbal medicated oils are available outside of India including dhanvantari, ashwagandha and mahanarayana oils. For readers interested in experiencing these oils, there is a list of suppliers in the Resources section at the end of this book.

177

Specific rejuvenating food, herbs and tonics

In Ayurveda, certain foods and herbs have long been recognised as having rejuvenating properties. Foods such as almonds, dates, figs, milk, ghee and medicinal herbs such as ashwagandha (*Withania somnifera*), shatavari (*Asparagus racemosa*), amalaki (*Emblica officianalis*) and brahmi (*Bacopa monnieri*) are some examples. Various kinds of tonics are used to strengthen specific organs in the body and facilitate an additional level of nourishment. I include here some tonics that can be made at home and are easy to prepare.

Date shake

6 dates, pitted
1½ cups milk
½ teaspoon vanilla extract
½ cup shredded coconut

Place all ingredients in a blender and process until smooth. Serve immediately. *Note*: Vata-predominant body types may like to add a pinch of cardamom to increase the digestibility of this drink.

Fig shake

3 dried figs
1½ cups apple juice
1 teaspoon almond meal
1 pinch ground cloves

Place all ingredients in a blender and process until smooth. Serve immediately.

Rejuvenating almond milk

5 almonds soaked overnight in a cup of water
1 cup of milk
½ teaspoon of ground cardamom

Drain almonds and peel them. (The skin is largely indigestible.) In a small saucepan bring milk to the boil. Pour hot milk, almonds and cardamom into a blender and process until smooth. Serve immediately.

Rasayana for the weary

The recipe for this rejuvenating tonic was given to me by my friend, Tim Mitchell, and was passed onto him by his teacher, who in turn received it from his teacher. It can serve as an excellent meal replacement, especially late in the evening, when having a full meal would be too much. It is easy to digest and particularly nourishing.

5–10 saffron threads
2 tablespoons hot water
1 cup milk (organic, unhomogenised)
½–2 teaspoons raw honey
½–2 teaspoons ghee

Soak the saffron threads in the hot water for 5–10 minutes, then add them and the water to the cup of milk. Bring the mixture to the boil in a small saucepan. When the milk begins to froth, remove the saucepan from the heat. Wait 30 seconds until froth has settled and then bring the mixture to the boil again. Repeat this procedure once more so that the mixture has boiled three times. This process makes the milk lighter and easier to digest. Remove the saucepan from the heat and allow the mixture to cool to a lukewarm temperature. If you like you can do this by pouring the mixture from cup to cup.

When the mixture is lukewarm, add unequal amounts of ghee and honey. (Equal amounts of honey and ghee are said to create toxicity in Ayurvedic texts and are therefore avoided.) I include here a few possible combinations that can be used depending on how you are feeling and what your intuition is telling you.

½ teaspoon honey to 1 teaspoon ghee

1 teaspoon honey to 2 teaspoons ghee

1 teaspoon honey to ½ teaspoon ghee

2 teaspoons honey to 1 teaspoon ghee

Finally the instruction is to stir the contents of the cup in a clockwise direction. You are also advised to drink the tonic quickly and not sip it.

Rejuvenating tonic for sexual depletion

1 cup milk

2 teaspoons fresh ginger, grated

2 teaspoons white or black sesame seeds

2 teaspoons ghee

1 pinch cinnamon

honey to taste, if desired

Warm milk to a comfortable temperature. Blend all ingredients in a blender. Can be drunk daily as a sexual restorative or after sex, especially by men.

Rejuvenating Ayurvedic medicinal herbs

Within the herbal tradition of Ayurveda, there are a number of herbs that have been found to have a rejuvenating effect on the body-mind. They are known as tonic herbs because they help to build up the quality and quantity of certain tissues in the body. They tend to have a sweet taste and a heavy, oily quality.

I include here four popular rejuvenating medicinal herbs that are useful in restoring vitality to organs in the body that have become depleted in the context of chronic stress. This stress may be physical, emotional, mental or spiritual and is often a combination of these four kinds of stress. You will see that the four different herbs have affinities with different parts of the body, which they are known to specifically nourish.

Amalaki (Indian gooseberry) is one of the strongest rejuvenatives used in Ayurveda. The fruit is sour and is one of the highest sources of vitamin C, with 3000 mg per fruit. It is particularly effective for the blood, bones, liver and heart. It cleanses the intestines and regulates blood sugar. The part used is the fruit. It is the basis for Chyavan Prash, a medicated jam much prized in India, which is a good all-round tonic and restorative. It can be bought at Indian spice shops and is available online. I include some reputable herbal companies in the Resources section at the end of this book that sell good quality Ayurvedic herbal products, including Chyavan Prash.

Brahmi (Indian pennywort) is particularly revitalising for the nerves and the brain cells. It has been researched in Australia and abroad and has been found to be useful in enhancing cognitive function in the elderly. In Ayurveda it is said to increase intelligence and memory, and decrease senility and ageing. Brahmi is a powerful blood purifier and is useful in chronic skin diseases such as eczema and psoriasis. It has a calming effect on the nerves and can be taken as a tea before meditation. The part used is the leaf.

Ashwagandha (winter cherry) is one of the best rejuvenative herbs for the muscles, bone marrow and semen. It is used in cases of nervous exhaustion and weakness and when there is debilitation from chronic disease. Overwork, lack of sleep and adrenal depletion are all indications for the use of Ashwagandha. It helps to build up tissue in the body and slow the ageing process. It has a nurturing effect on the mind and helps promote deep, restful sleep. The part used is the root.

Shatavari (wild asparagus) is the main rejuvenative herb used in Ayurveda for the female reproductive system. It is very soothing and nourishing for dry and inflamed mucus membranes of the lungs, stomach, kidneys and sexual organs. It increases milk and semen and is excellent in the treatment of menopause. It nourishes the female ovum and increases fertility. The part used is the root.

My journey of rejuvenation

I include this account of the experiences of a patient of mine, Tanya, who was referred to me by a general practitioner colleague for help in managing long-term stress.

Sadly, I was a regular visitor to my GP's clinic with constant colds, viruses and sore throats, along with some depression and anxiety. I was in overdrive, working long hours, travelling and struggling to be a decent mother to my beautiful three-year-old son. I was concerned about my health. I knew that if I continued like this I was heading towards a serious life-threatening illness.

After one consult with my Ayurvedic doctor the fears started to ease. I was given a 20-minute daily meditation and an Ayurvedic herb by the name of ashwaghanda to balance my Vata dosha and nervous system. I started to feel calmer. I wanted more of this, and I knew I was on the right path.

My next leap of faith was on my doctor's suggestion to do a seven-day rejuvenation program at an Ayurvedic resort called Isola di Coco, located in Kerala, India. I dove in and booked my trip within a week.

So there I was, on my own, in India, frazzled, apprehensive, and ready for a change.

On the first day, I had a consult with the resort Ayurvedic doctor and then it was time for my treatments to begin. Being coated and massaged in warm oil infused with medicinal plants and herbs by locally trained therapists was just out of this world. After three hours of several types of oil treatments I staggered back to my room and fell into a deep, luxurious slumber.

For seven life-changing days I practised morning yoga and meditations with a local swami. Steaming pots of cumin and ginger teas along with delicious Ayurvedic vegetarian meals tailored to my dosha type built up my fragile system. With each mouthful I knew I was being healed.

My days were spent having various oil treatments such as shirodhara to ease the headaches and mental tension. Kizhi pouch massage relieved my aches and pains. Herbal powder body scrubs removed toxins and fat. My skin became radiant from the facials concocted of fresh orange, cucumbers, and milk and fruit pastes.

The extra weight was falling away, my skin and eyes glowed, I felt alive, energised and well again. By day five, I was bounding out of bed. Now that hadn't happened in a long, long time.

Upon my return, friends and family remarked on the change – physical, mental and spiritual. I felt it and I knew that this was the way for me to have a healthy and happy life.

> *It was then that I made a vow to myself to return each year to Kerala to rejuvenate, and I have done so.*
>
> *That was over four years ago and the power of Ayurveda has never left me. I do fall off the wagon sometimes, but through the knowledge of Ayurveda, I have made courageous changes to my lifestyle, found my joy and have these ancient tools to heal and rejuvenate.*

Creating institutions that support ageing

One of my challenges as an educator is to try to successfully integrate the principles of these ancient wisdom traditions into a modern, Western context. When it comes to the subject of how to care for the elderly, it is important to acknowledge the inherent differences between traditional cultures (based around living with one's extended family), and modern, Western culture (where we tend to live with our nuclear family, as separate individuals or as a couple).

When someone loses their capacity to live independently here in the West, they are often forced to seek the support of an institution such as a hostel or nursing home in order to carry on. In this context, creating institutions that can best meet that person's physical, emotional, mental, social and spiritual needs is of paramount importance. It has been my good fortune to witness firsthand the workings of a modern aged-care facility that has been able to honour the needs of its clients and patients in just such ways. An institution committed to creating an environment where its residents are cared for humanely, and which enables them to live with dignity.

The facility of which I speak is best described as a campus that has been purpose-built by a Jewish organisation to meet the needs of the local Jewish community. It is well resourced and well run and receives generous donations from wealthy benefactors. What becomes obvious after a short time is the extent to which the facility is integrated into the local Jewish community on lots of levels.

The central point of the campus is a large, open-style lounge come recreational space, where relatives can enjoy a cup of coffee or tea with their family members. The lounge is close to the hostel area, where residents live independently, and the higher dependency wards, where residents with dementia or chronic, debilitating medical conditions live. It also serves as a place where people can play cards, read newspapers and connect with staff working in the facility. What emerges is a friendly and inclusive atmosphere that sets the tone for the whole establishment.

Once a week a group of 20 or so children from a nearby Jewish preschool visit the facility with their teachers. It is extraordinary how much joy they bring to the residents as they wander noisily through the wards, hostel areas and coffee lounge. Old faces come to life and engage beautifully with the children, who seem to take it all in their stride. After school hours, high school students from a local Jewish school can often be seen sitting with residents listening to stories from their lives with rapt attention. Additionally, there is a strong volunteer presence in the campus that lends warmth and goodwill to the overall mix.

The facility has a number of gardens in the complex, some of which adjoin the closed wards where residents with dementia are housed. Recognising the importance of having regular contact with nature, each week, weather permitting, diversion therapists hold groups amongst the shrubs and trees. The larger open garden is also well used by independently living residents who can often be seen catching up with their family members and friends under the judiciously placed umbrellas and benches. The principle of using natural surroundings to support healing and rejuvenation, which has long been recognised in Ayurveda, is certainly put to good use in the complex.

THE PRINCIPLE OF USING NATURAL SURROUNDINGS TO SUPPORT HEALING AND REJUVENATION, WHICH HAS LONG BEEN RECOGNISED IN AYURVEDA, IS PUT TO GOOD USE ...

Another aspect of the service and care provided to residents is the management's commitment to the maintenance of Jewish religious and cultural traditions. The ancient Jewish holy days and festivals are honoured throughout the year and pains are also taken to explain their significance and help residents and families connect with their traditions. Each Friday evening Shabbat ceremonies are conducted by visiting rabbis in a number of different wards, enabling residents to draw comfort and peace of mind from this shared religious experience. The friendly and inclusive way in which it is held allows both Jewish and non-Jewish residents and their relatives to feel that they are part of a big family. The excitement and happiness this occasion generates in the residents, some of whom are struggling with dementia, is always touching to behold.

Not being Jewish myself, it has been a real eye-opener to see the many ways in which this aged-care facility supports and is supported by the local Jewish community. It not only offers first-rate care of the elderly and infirm members of its community, but it has become a fundamental pillar in the lives of many families, enabling a remarkable level of social cohesion and connectedness in the midst of a large and multicultural city such as Sydney.

At the end of your life

Although you cannot predict the circumstances of your own death, whether it takes place in a hospice, hospital, at home or in an accident, you are able to prepare for that time throughout your life. From a Buddhist perspective, living well and dying well are seen as two sides of the same coin, the idea that the best preparation for your inevitable death is to have lived a life well lived. A life where you have expressed yourself fully in the various domains of your life that now allows you to embrace its passing.

For many people, death and the fear of the unknown is frightening. For even more, dying painfully and with a loss of dignity and control is a much larger fear. So how can we come to a place where we can face our death and the dying process with openness and acceptance?

A proactive approach to your death and the dying process is a powerful starting point. To be actively involved in the enquiry into who dies and to develop the kind of internal resources required to be open to the experience of dying is a prerequisite in my view.

This is where the place of spiritual practices that allow you to connect with your essential nature is invaluable. Naturally those practices will reflect your spiritual orientation during your life, whether coming from a specific religious tradition or from your own personal belief system. From the perspective of yoga, your true identity is timeless and changeless, unencumbered by your physical body. Through earnest enquiry supported by spiritual practices, it is possible to move this kind of understanding from an intellectual acceptance to a much deeper knowing of the heart. Once you realise that you are, in essence, the deathless spirit, the occurrence of your death loses its significance.

Spiritual practices that align you with your spiritual nature during your lifetime can help you surrender to the experience of dying. This is where having some facility in meditation can put you in good stead as you embark on the process of letting go to the great unknown.

We are fortunate in the present age to be able, for the most part, to relieve the distressing symptoms of terminal illness using modern medicines. Meditation and healing practices such as massage, reflexology, Reiki and sound therapy can also help people deal with unpleasant symptoms such as pain and nausea. They can also allow you to retain a greater sense of control in the dying process.

Through their ability to help you connect with your inner stillness, these practices can also relieve the anxiety, guilt and anger that sometimes arises at the end of your life. By staying more connected to the big picture, rather than the roller-coaster of your thoughts and emotions, a more calm and grounded state of mind becomes possible. Naturally, this can help support the process of saying goodbye to partners, family members and friends, as we prepare for our death.

... THE PREPARATION FOR YOUR DEATH IS REALLY JUST ANOTHER PART OF YOUR ENQUIRY INTO LIFE ...

On a practical level, taking time to prepare your will and funeral instructions is a very useful process and while confronting, supports you in facing your death. One patient of mine, a woman in quite reasonable health in her seventies, designed her coffin and then had it built in preparation for her death. She lives an active life as an artist, but wants to embrace the last part of her life. Making sure the financial arrangements after your passing are satisfying to you is also important, so that the needs of those closest to you are taken into consideration and looked after.

In these ways, the preparation for your death is really just another part of your enquiry into life – nothing more, nothing less. It becomes a vehicle for your journey of understanding into what is changeless in life and what continues after your body dies.

Rejuvenation as a way of being

In this chapter we have looked at various approaches to restore vitality and wellbeing using ancient principles of preventive medicine and specific rejuvenating therapies. This is a path through life where you learn to travel lightly, thereby creating less wear and tear on the body. Through an attentive listening to your body, you learn how to better manage and conserve your energy. In simple terms, you learn how to prevent yourself becoming depleted and how to renew yourself if you do. Necessarily this involves wiser choices around your diet and lifestyle, prioritising your health needs and developing a network of practitioners with different skills to support your personal wellbeing. Practitioners who can help you with your diet, teach you yoga and meditation practices, give you a revitalising oil massage or reflexology treatment or support you in working through a challenging emotional predicament.

As we have seen, there are specific foods and herbs that are known for their rejuvenation properties, as well as practices of self-care that nourish debilitated organs in the body. As these practices become integrated into your life, your moment-to-moment awareness of yourself and your environment goes through a profound transformation. Essentially what emerges is a way of being in the world that is both sustaining and sustainable. A way of being that equips you well for the long haul and which supports you in ageing gracefully.

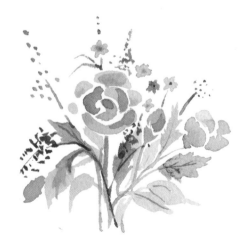

Conclusion

While running an Ayurvedic cooking class many years ago, I happened to meet a young woman in her mid-twenties who had volunteered to assist my co-teacher and me. It turned out that she was an aspiring actress and was now in the process of auditioning for parts in the theatre, television and film industry. She had an interest in natural therapies and had recently completed a three-year course in naturopathy. During the day she shared with me, 'When I finished high school I realised that I needed to learn how to look after myself and studying natural therapies helped me do that.' More aware of her physical, emotional, mental and spiritual health needs and how to support them, she now felt equipped to follow her real calling as an actress.

I was impressed by her wise approach and wondered why this kind of knowledge has not traditionally been taught in schools. Fortunately some in-roads have been made on this front as personal development, health and wellbeing courses are now available in many secondary schools. That said, it would be heartening to see some of the principles explored in this book become available to young people to help them prepare for their lives after school.

The approaches to the art of balanced living presented in these pages were developed many thousands of years ago. However, when modified for time and context, they are as relevant today as they were in the past. Essentially they provide a framework that can give us direction as we navigate through life; a framework that allows for our intuition and the guidance that can come from this dimension of our experience.

They are approaches that encourage connection with ourselves, with our fellow human beings and with the natural world. By broadening our awareness of ourselves and the effects of our actions, they support a way of being that reminds us that we are all a small part of a complex web of relationships.

What is apparent from the personal stories shared in this book is that there are already people from all walks of life drawing from these traditions of wellbeing.

Through cultivating more balance in their lives, they are reaping the rewards in terms of greater satisfaction and more joy in their everyday experience.

The benefits they are experiencing flow into the lives of their families, friends, workmates and their communities. It is timely that these traditions find their rightful place in our global discourse on how best to move forward, given the personal, social and environmental challenges of the 21st century. It is my sincere hope that this book may help bridge the current divide that exists between mainstream Western culture and these ancient traditions of wellbeing and graceful living.

Grace

The basic premise that underpins the wisdom traditions presented in this book is that your essential nature is peace. The St James Bible describes it beautifully as 'the peace that passeth all understanding'. It's a peace that is with you all the time whatever challenges and struggles you may be facing. It is simply obscured by the machinations of your mind, like a cloud that keeps the sun hidden from view.

These ancient approaches to wellbeing, when lived, help you to stay connected to your innate stillness and inner knowing. Importantly, they are oral traditions that involve being part of a teacher–student relationship, based on mutual respect. The guidance of a qualified teacher, in tandem with your personal practice, allows the richness of these traditions to flower and bear fruit in your life. It is through the practice of these principles that you make them your own.

In the beginning, an act of faith is required, as some of these principles may seem quite foreign for people who have grown up in the West. But, in my experience, and certainly the experience of many of my students and colleagues, is that faith will be well rewarded.

A process of refinement takes place whereby you begin to manage your energy with more and more awareness by asking such questions as, 'How am I feeling in my body after this meal? How has that yoga practice affected my mood? How is my day different when I give myself some quality time in the morning? What is the quality of my thoughts after I meditate?'

This line of enquiry helps you to stay more in tune with yourself and how you are travelling through the day. With this knowledge, you can then make small changes to your diet, lifestyle and frame of mind to help you feel more balanced from moment to moment. Over time, the way you approach life is subtly, but powerfully, transformed.

Taking some time each day to focus on spiritual practices that connect you with your essential nature is paramount in this process of refinement. Practices that quieten the mind, enliven your senses and deliver you into the simplicity of the present moment. When you're feeling nourished on many levels, gratitude quite naturally arises, and with it a deep desire to contribute in some way to the welfare of our planet and the beings with which we share it. A gratitude for all the things that life has given you, the hard times as well as the good times. In those moments when the heart is full, the whole process of life is embraced, just as it is.

It is then that you are open to the grace that is your birthright, a grace that has always been working its magic and is always with you. With that sense of grace comes contentment that values the simple things in life and is not swayed by the 'slings and arrows of outrageous fortune'. An ancient Indian text states that, 'Contentment is the ultimate wealth'. Contentment that runs as a silent undercurrent in your life, which can be a source of perennial nourishment.

Appendices

Appendix 1:
Meal plans for the three body types

The following suggestions are a useful starting point. With practice you can modify and refine them after observing how the meals affect you and by using your intuition. I have included a few recipes that will be unfamiliar to many Westerners; keep in mind that a little trust can go a long way! Note that meals with one asterisk (*) can be found in Appendix 2.

Vata meals for summer

Breakfast

Seasonal sweet and juicy fruit (such as mango, papaya, stone fruits)

Toast with tahini, almond paste or avocado

Toasted muesli

Eggs on toast

Lunch

Upma*

Khichari*

Dahl* or seasonal mixed vegetables* and rice/quinoa/millet

Dinner

Soup (using root vegetables including carrot and parsnip with miso as stock)

Salad (rocket, avocado, lettuce, tomato) with tuna or pan-fried haloumi strips

Beverages

Herbal teas – chamomile, mint, green, bancha (twig), Vata-pacifying tea*

Vata meals for winter

Breakfast

Oatmeal porridge

Apple and millet*

Semolina halva*

Stewed fruit (apples, pears, stone fruit)
    with a pinch of cinnamon

Eggs on toast

Lunch

Khichari*

Dahl* and rice/quinoa/millet

Okra or green bean karhi*

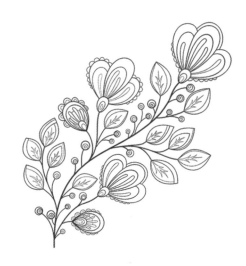

Dinner

Soup (pumpkin, sweet potato, miso and vegetables) and flat bread (chippati, roti) or toast
or rasam* or tofu mulligatawny soup*

Upma*

Beverages

Chai*, miso broth, green, chamomile, gotu cola tea

Pitta meals for summer

Breakfast

Fresh fruit in season, avoiding sour fruits (such as grapefruit)

Muesli (toasted/untoasted)

Toast with fruit toppings or avocado

Eggs on toast (occasionally)

Lunch

Salad with leafy greens, avocado, radicchio with butter/lima beans or tuna

Lisa's Byron Bay Salad*

Gado gado*

Dinner

Vegetarian salad

Seasonal mixed vegetables* and basmati rice

Beverages

Mint tea, coconut water, Pitta-pacifying tea, lassi,
black tea with milk

Pitta meals for winter

Breakfast

Oatmeal porridge

Berry muffins*

Quinoa treat*

Apple and millet*

Eggs on toast

Toast with fruit toppings, avocado

Lunch

Khichari* and flat bread (chapatti, roti)

Bean Provençal*

Baked ricotta*

Dinner

Soup

Seasonal mixed Vegetables* and rice/millet/quinoa

Spinach dahl*

Beverages

Pitta-reducing tea, mint tea, agni tea, gotu cola, green tea, black tea with/without milk

Kapha meals for summer

Breakfast

Puffed millet, amaranth with fresh fruit (strawberry, grated apple, berries)

Toast with bitter marmalade

Lunch

Khichari*

Seasonal mixed vegetables* with barley, millet/quinoa

Pauwa* (savoury puffed rice)

Beetroot curry*

Gado gado*

Dinner

Light salad (bitter greens, radicchio, sprouts) with spicy dressing

Spicy soup

Rasam*

Beverages

Kapha-pacifying tea, ginger tea, green tea, chai without milk

Kapha menu for winter

Breakfast

Spiced oatmeal porridge with cinnamon/cloves/ginger

Buckwheat pancakes*

Stewed fruit (apple, strawberry)

Apple and millet*

Lunch

Spinach dahl* and basmati rice/millet/quinoa

Khichari* with corn tortilla/chips

Spicy potatoes*

Tofu and vegetable stir-fry

Dinner

Rasam* with rye crackers

Spicy soup with rice crackers

Lime pickles or chutney

Steamed vegetables and rice/millet/quinoa

Beverages

Kapha-pacifying tea, ginger tea,
green tea, chai without milk

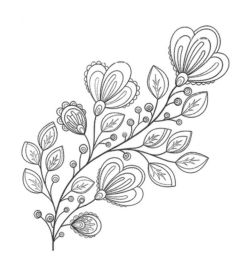

Appendix 2:
Recipes to pacify Vata, Pitta and Kapha dosha

The following are recipes for breakfast, lunch and dinner for each of the three body types. The recipes can also be used to pacify the dosha you feel is out of balance at the time of cooking. Many of these recipes were demonstrated at the Ayurvedic cooking classes I taught with my friend Tim Mitchell, a gifted Ayurvedic cook, in Sydney over almost two decades.

Vata-pacifying recipes

Apple and millet breakfast

A warm, nourishing breakfast that is easy to digest, alkalising and protein-rich. It favours sweet, sour and salty tastes, making it ideal for people with a Vata body type.

> 2 apples (Delicious, Pink Lady or Fuji), cut into 2-cm (¾ inch) cubes
> ½ cup hulled organic millet
> ¼ cup sultanas
> ¼ teaspoon cinnamon powder
> 1 pinch Celtic sea salt
> 1 teaspoon ghee or olive oil
> cold water

- Place all ingredients in a saucepan with enough water so that the top of the mixture is 2 cm below the surface of the water. Bring to the boil.
- Turn down to a low heat and let simmer with saucepan lid on until most of the water is absorbed, approx. 15–20 minutes. Once water is mostly absorbed, turn off the heat, cover and let sit for 5 minutes.
- Serve warm with a cup of your favourite breakfast tea.

Okra in yoghurt sauce (okra karhi)

One of the most popular dishes at our Ayurvedic cooking classes. It's a great way to experiment with okra for those not used to cooking with this interesting vegetable, which is very easy to digest.

2 cups okra (lady's fingers) or green beans

1 tablespoon ghee or sunflower oil

1 tablespoon mustard seeds

1 teaspoon cumin seeds

½ teaspoon turmeric powder

3 tablespoons chickpea (besan) flour

2 cups water

2 cups yoghurt

3 tablespoons lime juice

1 teaspoon brown sugar or rice syrup

1 teaspoon Celtic sea salt

freshly chopped coriander, to serve

rice, or other grain, to serve

- ◉ Wash and dry okra then cut off the tops. Heat ghee or oil in a large saucepan and add mustard and cumin seeds. When mustard seeds pop and cumin seeds are a darker shade of brown, add the okra and dust with turmeric. Cover and cook gently for 5 minutes, shaking the pan often.
- ◉ Combine chickpea flour, water and yoghurt in a large bowl. Whisk until a smooth consistency is reached. Add this yoghurt mixture to the okra and spices with the remaining ingredients.
- ◉ Cook for 20 minutes over a low to medium heat, stirring occasionally. Garnish with freshly chopped coriander and serve with your favourite grain.

Beetroot soup (borscht)

A hearty beetroot soup that makes for a wonderful winter warmer.

1 large potato, thinly sliced

2 large beetroots, thinly sliced

1 vegetarian stock cube

4–6 cups water

1 large onion, chopped

2 tablespoons ghee or olive oil

½ teaspoon caraway seeds

¼ teaspoon dill seeds

¼ teaspoon black pepper

2 teaspoons Celtic sea salt

1 large carrot, sliced

1 stalk celery, chopped

3 cups chopped cabbage

1 tablespoon raisins

1 tablespoon apple cider vinegar

½ cup tomato puree

sour cream, to serve

dill, finely chopped, to serve

- Place potato, beets, stock cube and water in a large saucepan and cook vegetables until tender. Drain, reserving water.
- In a large frying pan, cook the onions in ghee or oil and add the spices, pepper and salt. Cook onion until translucent and then add carrot, celery and cabbage.
- Add the water from the beets and potatoes and cook until all the vegetables are tender.
- Add the potatoes, beets and remaining ingredients. Cover and simmer on a low heat for 30 minutes. Serve with sour cream and fresh dill.

Tofu mulligatawny soup

A stalwart dish at our autumn Ayurvedic cooking classes that is perfect when you're feeling depleted and low in energy. Non-vegetarians may substitute chicken for tofu. It is very strengthening and nourishing for Vata imbalances.

500 g (1 lb) firm tofu cut into 2 cm (¾ inch) cubes

2 tablespoons ghee or olive oil

¼ teaspoon fenugreek seeds

4 cm (1½ inches) fresh ginger, finely chopped

2 cloves garlic, finely chopped

1 cinnamon quill

10 curry leaves

10 threads saffron

900 ml (30 fluid oz) water

300 ml (10 fluid oz) coconut milk

1 tablespoon coriander powder

1 tablespoon cumin powder

2 vegetable stock cubes

1 small onion, finely chopped

4 small tomatoes

1 lime, juiced

Celtic sea salt, according to taste

- Sauté tofu in 1 tablespoon of the ghee or oil in a large frying pan until browned. In a large saucepan, add remaining oil and sauté fenugreek, ginger, garlic, cinnamon, curry leaves and saffron gently before adding tofu cubes.
- In a large bowl, whisk together the water, coconut milk, coriander and cumin powders and add to the mixture in the saucepan along with the stock cubes. Simmer for 30 minutes.
- In the same frying pan used earlier, brown the chopped onion then stir in tomatoes. When softened, add to the soup. Season with lime juice and salt.

Vermicelli milk pudding (payasam)

This recipe was demonstrated to me by an Indian mother while I was staying at her family's Ayurvedic ashram in Kerala. Serve warm or cold depending on weather and inclination.

1 litre (33 fluid oz) milk

1 cup wheat vermicelli, broken into 6 cm pieces

3 tablespoons ghee

1 pinch saffron

⅓ teaspoon ground cardamom

½ cup cashews

½ cup sultanas

1 cup sugar

- Slowly bring milk to boil over low heat, stirring well.
- Gently fry vermicelli in 2 tablespoons of the ghee, turning continuously until golden brown. Let vermicelli cool and then rinse in water several times.
- Once milk has boiled, add vermicelli, saffron and cardamom.
- Gently fry cashews and sultanas in leftover ghee.
- Add sugar to milk mixture and then cashews and sultanas, stirring continuously for a minimum of 10 minutes. Cover pot and let sit until ready to serve.

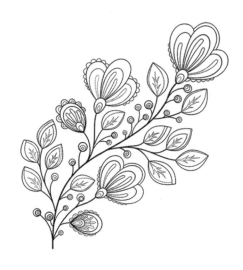

Pitta-pacifying recipes

Martin's quinoa treat

This recipe comes from a friend of mine who runs a popular vegetarian restaurant in Darwin. Customers travel from all over the Northern Territory to partake of this dish. It combines all six tastes described in Ayurveda, making it a well-balanced meal. A mouth-watering breakfast or dessert all year round.

1 kg (2 lbs) pears, diced

¾ cup quinoa (half red and half white)

300 ml (10 fluid oz) coconut milk

1 tablespoon cinnamon powder

3 star anise

500 ml (16 fluid oz) water

¼ cup grated ginger

200 g (7 oz) fresh dates

1 fresh lime, juiced

full-cream natural yoghurt and walnuts, to taste

⊙ Put all ingredients except lime, yoghurt and walnuts together in a large pot. Cook over medium heat for 20–30 minutes, stirring occasionally, until fruit is soft.

⊙ Add lime juice so you have a nice contrast of sweet, tangy and gingery tastes. Serve warm with a dollop of yoghurt and walnuts on top.

Lisa's Byron Bay salad

This was the most popular salad at a café in Byron Bay owned by a member of my extended family. It's a meal in itself that is brimming with flavour.

olive oil, Celtic sea salt and pepper

6 Roma tomatoes, halved

1 handful green beans, tops removed

1 handful snow peas, tops removed

250 g (½ lb) haloumi cheese, sliced into thin strips

1 tablespoon olive oil

½ bunch shallots

1 Spanish onion, finely chopped

½ bunch fresh dill, finely chopped

½ bunch fresh mint, finely chopped

1 handful kalamata olives

Dressing:

olive oil

balsamic vinegar

Celtic sea salt

freshly cracked pepper

- Preheat oven to 160°C. Brush each tomato with olive oil and then season with sea salt and cracked pepper. Place on an oven tray lined with baking paper to absorb moisture and slow roast for 1½ hours. Let cool and then cut in half again.
- Blanch green beans and snow peas, refresh under cold water, then cut in half.
- Pan-fry haloumi cheese in the olive oil until crisp and golden. Set aside.
- Place shallots, Spanish onion, dill, mint, green beans, snow peas and olives in a bowl.
- To make dressing, mix together half balsamic vinegar, half olive oil, ground Celtic sea salt and cracked pepper. Drizzle over salad and toss just before serving.

Gado gado (an Indonesian salad delight)

250 g (½ lb) bok choy

125 g (¼ lb) mung bean shoots

1 handful green beans

450 g (1 lb) tofu, cut into 2-cm cubes

sesame oil for deep frying

½ medium cucumber, cut into batons

1 small bunch watercress

1 tablespoon fresh lime juice

black pepper to taste

Dressing:

chilli powder

¾ cup dry-roasted peanuts (or almonds, if allergic to peanuts)

1 teaspoon Celtic sea salt

1 teaspoon brown sugar or jaggary

250 ml (8 fluid oz) cold water

½ cup coconut milk

- Blanch the bok choy in boiling water for one minute and drain well. Blanch bean shoots in the same way for 30 seconds. Cook green beans in lightly salted boiling water for 5 minutes.
- Deep fry tofu in sesame oil until golden and then drain.
- To make the dressing, place chilli powder, dry-roasted nuts, salt and sugar into a blender or food processer. Blend into a smooth powder, then add cold water to the mix. Transfer contents to a heavy pan and bring to the boil, then simmer for 5 minutes. Add the coconut milk and remove from the heat.
- Make artful piles of bok choy, bean shoots, green beans, cucumber, tofu cubes and watercress on each individual plate.
- Reheat the dressing, add lime juice and mix well then pour over the salad. Serve immediately.

Mixed vegetables in coconut milk (aviyal)

3 tablespoons raw cashews

3 tablespoons ghee

1 pinch asafoetida

2 tablespoons fresh ginger, grated

6–8 fresh curry leaves

2–3 cups mixed vegetables (eg carrots, green beans, kumera, cauliflower)

1 teaspoon sweet chilli sauce

½ teaspoon turmeric powder

400 ml (14 fluid oz) coconut milk

1–2 teaspoons Celtic sea salt

10 snow peas

rice, or your favourite grain, to serve

- Gently roast the cashews in ghee in a large frying pan, tossing often to prevent burning. Remove the cashews and set aside.
- Add to the remaining ghee the asafoetida, ginger and curry leaves, frying gently. Increase the heat and add the mixed vegetables, sweet chilli sauce, turmeric powder and coconut milk. Season with sea salt and simmer for 10–15 minutes until tender.
- Remove the frying pan from the stove and place the snow peas on top of the mixture, then add the roasted cashews. Replace the lid and wait 5 minutes for the food to settle.
- Stir and serve with your favourite grain.

Timbeau's baked ricotta

A vegetarian Sunday roast that beautifully complements a vegetable and rice dish. Very popular with children and great in sandwiches the next day.

1 teaspoon tarragon leaves

1 teaspoon paprika

½ teaspoon turmeric

freshly ground black pepper, to taste

4 tablespoons olive or macadamia oil

½ teaspoon Celtic sea salt

375 g (13 oz) fresh ricotta slice or slab

◉ Preheat oven to 180°C (350° Fahrenheit).

◉ Mix together the tarragon leaves, spices, pepper, oil and sea salt in a small bowl.

◉ Place the ricotta slab on an oiled tray and baste with the herb and spiced oil.

◉ Bake in oven for about 45 minutes, basting several times throughout.

◉ When lightly browned, remove from oven and allow to cool a little before cutting to serve.

Bean Provençale

A quick and easy dish using Western culinary herbs that is ideal for people with a Pitta body type. It is tasty, but is not overly heating.

1 tablespoon olive oil
1 large onion, sliced
1 small red capsicum, sliced
1 small green capsicum, sliced
1 clove garlic, crushed
3 teaspoons tomato paste
fresh basil and oregano leaves, chopped
½ cup water
⅓ cup pitted black olives
¼ bunch parsley, chopped
3 ripe tomatoes, chopped
1 x 440 g (16 oz) can four-bean mix, drained
couscous or rice, to serve
1 handful of chopped parsley, to serve

- Heat oil in large frying pan and stir-fry onion for approximately 2 minutes. Add capsicum and garlic and fry for a further 3 minutes.
- Add remaining ingredients and cook on medium heat, stirring regularly, until ingredients are well mixed into a stew. Let bubble on low heat as time allows.
- Turn off heat and let sit for a few minutes. Serve over couscous or rice and garnish with a little parsley.

'Berry good' muffins

1¼ cups unbleached wholemeal flour

1 cup barley flour

¾ cup raw sugar

2 teaspoons baking powder

⅓ cup sunflower oil

1 cup plain yoghurt

2 eggs

¼ cup milk (or rice or almond milk)

1½ cups blueberries or raspberries

Topping:

1 tablespoon raw sugar

1 teaspoon cinnamon powder

2 tablespoons almond flakes

- Preheat oven to 200°C (375° Fahrenheit) and grease a 12-hole muffin tray.
- Mix flour, sugar and baking powder together.
- In a separate bowl, beat together the oil, yoghurt, eggs and milk until light and fluffy. Gently mix together the wet and dry ingredients so that the mixture is moist and lumpy. Fold in the berries gently, mixing minimally.
- Mix together the sugar, cinnamon and almond flakes to make the topping. Scoop batter into muffin tray, filling each to three-quarters full, and sprinkle with the topping.
- Bake for 20–25 minutes. Cool for 10 minutes before serving.

Kapha-pacifying recipes

Buckwheat pancakes

1½ cups buckwheat flour

½ cup oat bran

1 teaspoon baking powder

1 pinch cinnamon powder

½ teaspoon Celtic sea salt

1 egg

1½ cups plain yoghurt

1½ cups water

2 teaspoons sunflower oil

honey, maple syrup or your favourite berry, to serve

⊚ Mix together all the dry ingredients in a large bowl. In another bowl, beat the egg, yoghurt, water and oil. Add the liquid mixture to the dry mixture, stirring minimally.

⊚ Pour onto a hot, oiled frying pan. When bubbles appear on the edges of the pancake and underside is light brown, turn over. Place on individual plates and serve with honey, maple syrup or berries.

Spicy south Indian tomato consommé (rasam)

2 tablespoons tamarind pulp

1 cup of boiling water

2 tablespoons toor dal (yellow split peas) or red lentils

½ teaspoon turmeric powder

6 cups water

2 medium-sized tomatoes, diced

2 teaspoons rasam powder (available from Indian spice shops)

½ teaspoon jaggary (available from Indian spice shops)

1 teaspoon Celtic sea salt

1 tablespoon ghee

1 teaspoon brown mustard seeds

10 fresh curry leaves

½ teaspoon asafoetida

1 handful finely chopped coriander leaves, to serve

- Soak the tamarind in boiling water in a ceramic bowl.
- In a medium-sized saucepan, bring to the boil the dal or lentils, turmeric and water. Reduce the heat and simmer for 25 minutes. Whisk the ingredients at the end of the cooking process to encourage softening. Add the tomatoes, rasam powder, jaggary, sea salt and tamarind paste.
- In a small frying pan, heat the ghee and fry the mustard seeds until they turn grey. Add the curry leaves and cook until they turn dark green and start to crisp. Next add the asafoetida and cook for a few seconds before pouring all the cooked spices into the dahl pot.
- Cover the pot immediately, remove from the heat and set aside for 5–10 minutes before serving. Garnish with fresh coriander leaves.

Savoury flattened rice (pauwa)

A very quick breakfast dish or snack that needs minimal cooking once the potatoes have been boiled. It fulfils the Ayurvedic requirement of including all six tastes.

1 potato

1–2 teaspoons ghee or sesame oil

1 onion, chopped

1–2 green chillis

1 teaspoon turmeric powder

2 tablespoons brown mustard seeds

1 handful fresh curry leaves

1 cinnamon quill

1 teaspoon raw sugar

1 teaspoon Celtic sea salt

250 g (8 oz) pauwa (flattened rice), available from Indian spice shops

1 lime, juiced

1 small bunch fresh coriander leaves, finely chopped, to serve

- Boil potato, chop into small cubes and set aside.
- Heat ghee in a medium-sized wok or frying pan and sauté the onion; do not make it brown. Add potato cubes and then the chopped chilies, turmeric, mustard seeds, curry leaves, cinnamon, sugar and sea salt.
- Wash the rice in a sieve, drain and then add to the mixture in the wok. If necessary, wet it with a little water to make sure it does not dry up totally. Cover and steam for a few minutes. Pour the fresh lime juice over the rice and garnish with coriander leaves.

Spicy potatoes

2 tablespoons safflower oil

1 pinch asafoetida

1 teaspoon black mustard seeds

1 teaspoon cumin seeds

3 potatoes, peeled and cut into 2 cm (¾ inch) cubes

¼ teaspoon turmeric powder

½ teaspoon garam masala or cayenne pepper

½ teaspoon Celtic sea salt

2 tablespoons finely chopped coriander leaves, to serve

- Heat the oil in a frying pan until hot then add the asafoetida, mustard seeds and cumin seeds. Sauté until mustard seeds start to pop and cumin turns a darker shade of brown.
- Add the potatoes and dust with turmeric, masala powder and salt, stirring gently to ensure the potatoes are coated with spices.
- Cook over a low heat, covered, until tender, stirring every few minutes to prevent sticking. Garnish with fresh coriander leaves.

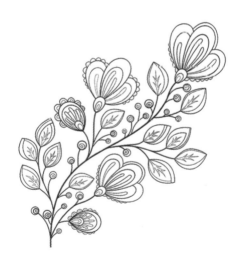

Beetroot curry

A Sri Lankan dish guaranteed to change your feeling for beetroot, if you are not already a true believer in this great root vegetable, which is rich in iron.

3–4 beetroots, sliced into large julienne shreds

1 tablespoons dry-roasted curry powder (Sri Lankan if possible)

1 tablespoon coriander powder

1 teaspoon turmeric powder

1 teaspoon Celtic sea salt

10 fresh curry leaves

1 can (300 ml/10 fluid oz) light coconut milk

300 ml (10 fluid oz) water

1 tablespoon safflower oil

1 pinch asafoetida

1 teaspoon fenugreek seeds

1 tablespoon cumin seeds

- Preheat oven to 180°C (350° Fahrenheit).
- In a large casserole dish, mix together the sliced beetroots, curry powder, coriander, turmeric, sea salt, curry leaves, coconut milk and water.
- In a small frying pan, heat the safflower oil, asafoetida, fenugreek and cumin seeds and fry for 1 minute.
- Add all the spices to the mixture in the casserole dish and stir well. Cover, then bake in oven for 1 hour.

Sweet potato halva

A very healthy dessert that uses no sugar, deriving its sweetness from the fruits, vegetables and spices used.

500 g (1 lb) sweet potato (kumera)
300 ml (10 fluid oz) milk
15 saffron threads
½ cup raisins
4 cardamom pods, crushed in a mortar
2 tablespoons ghee
½ cups slivered almonds

- Preheat oven to 180°C (350° Fahrenheit).
- Peel and grate the sweet potato.
- Bring the milk to the boil in a large frying pan, add the sweet potato and cook over medium heat for 15 minutes.
- Soak the saffron threads in a ¼ cup of hot water for 10 minutes. Stir the saffron and water, raisins, crushed cardamom and ghee and cook for another 10 minutes.
- Pour halva into a buttered dish, sprinkle with almonds and bake for 15 minutes. Serve with your favourite tea or chai.

Appendix 3:
Recipes to balance all three doshas

Semolina halva

A warm, sweet breakfast dish or snack that is easy to digest, cleansing and very nourishing.

> 1 cup coarse semolina
> 1 tablespoon ghee
> 2–3 cups water
> ½ cup rapadura sugar or jaggary (available from Indian spice shops)
> ½ cup almonds, chopped in half
> 1 cup sultanas and chopped dried apricots
> 1 teaspoon ground cardamom

- Gently roast the semolina in the ghee in a large frying pan over a low heat, constantly stirring until the semolina turns slightly brown and becomes aromatic.
- Add water to cover the grains and increase the heat to medium. Continue to stir to avoid the mixture becoming lumpy.
- Add rapadura sugar, nuts, dried fruit and cardamom and cook until all the liquid is absorbed. Turn off the heat.
- Cover the mixture and allow to stand for a further 10 minutes. Serve with your favourite tea or chai.

Upma

This is a popular savoury breakfast dish in south India, although it can be eaten any time. It uses semolina, which comes from the heart of wheat. Individuals with a gluten sensitivity can use polenta, made from corn, as a substitute. Upma is gently spiced and incorporates all six tastes making it appropriate for all body types.

1 cup coarse semolina

¼ cup ghee (Vatas and Pittas) or ¼ cup safflower oil (Kaphas)

1 pinch asafoetida

1 teaspoon black mustard seeds

1 teaspoon cumin seeds

2 cm fresh ginger, finely chopped

6 fresh curry leaves

½ teaspoon turmeric powder

1 small onion, finely chopped

½ cup coriander leaves, coarsely chopped

½ teaspoon Celtic sea salt

3 cups hot water, approximately

¼ cup shredded coconut, to serve

1 lime, to serve

- Gently dry roast semolina in a wok or frying pan on medium heat until slightly brown, stirring frequently. Set aside to cool.
- In a saucepan over medium heat, add ghee or oil. When ghee is hot, add asafoetida then mustard and cumin seeds. When mustard seeds pop, quickly stir in other spices, onion and half of the coriander leaves. Cook until onion is golden brown.
- Add roasted semolina and sea salt and mix well. Next, slowly pour in hot water, stirring the mixture to prevent lumps from forming. Simmer for a further 2 minutes, stirring continuously.
- Turn down heat to low and cover. Simmer for a further 5 minutes. Garnish with shredded coconut and remaining coriander leaves. Squeeze fresh lime over each serving.

Spinach dahl (Indian lentil soup)

1 cup mung dahl or red lentils

3–4 cups water

2 tablespoons ghee or favourite oil

2 teaspoons grated fresh ginger

1 teaspoon turmeric powder

1 bunch English spinach, finely chopped

1 pinch asafoetida

1 teaspoon mustard seeds

1 teaspoon cumin seeds

½ teaspoon ground black pepper

1 green chilli (optional, though Pitta types should refrain!)

1 lemon, juiced

Celtic sea salt

½ bunch of fresh coriander leaves, chopped

- Wash lentils well, at least three times. Add water until soup is as thick as you like it. Bring the mixture to a boil in a large saucepan. Scoop off froth and discard.
- Add 1 tablespoon of the ghee, ginger and turmeric powder and simmer over a low to medium heat for 30–40 minutes, stirring occasionally. Whisk the mixture to make a smooth, thick soup. Stir in spinach and keep on a gentle heat.
- Heat the remaining ghee in a small frying pan or spice skillet. Add asafoetida when the ghee is hot, then the mustard seeds until they pop, followed by the cumin and pepper. Carefully pour the spice mixture directly into the dahl and mix well.
- Stir in the lemon juice and salt and garnish with fresh coriander leaves. Cover and allow to settle for 5 minutes before serving.

Chai

Chai is a spiced, soothing Indian tea. There are many recipes for chai. Other spices to experiment with include nutmeg, cloves, peppercorns, fennel and star anise.

4 cups boiling water

3 cm (1¼ inch) fresh ginger, sliced

10 cardamom pods, bruised using a mortar and pestle

1 cinnamon quill

unprocessed sugar (rapadura, jaggary, palm or coconut sugar), according to taste

3–4 teaspoons (or tea bags) black tea (rooibos tea is caffeine free)

2 cups milk

⊙ In a large saucepan, bring water to the boil and add the spices above or those you have selected. Simmer for approximately 10 minutes to allow the spices to infuse through the water. Turn off the heat and allow the mixture to brew. Add the tea leaves or bags.

⊙ Bring the milk to the boil in a second saucepan and add to the tea and spice infusion. Gently simmer the mixture for a few more minutes, then remove from the heat and allow the ingredients to settle for another 5 minutes.

⊙ The ratio of water to milk can be adjusted for individual taste and the moment. Many people like a ratio of two parts of water to one part milk. This tea is also delicious without milk, which may suit people with more Kapha in their body type or those who are intolerant of dairy.

Thermos flask lunch

This recipe is a godsend for people who are heading off to work and are sick of eating takeaway food at lunchtime. All you need is an open-mouthed thermos flask, ten minutes in the morning and a Saturday to collect the required ingredients.

Everything is cooked in a small saucepan for 2–5 minutes and poured steaming hot into the thermos flask. With practice, the whole process can be completed in less than ten minutes and you get to enjoy a freshly cooked meal at lunchtime. The recipe can be modified for all three doshas and the seasons, as per the directions below, although this is just a starting point for your own creativity and intuition.

1 tablespoon olive oil or ghee

1 pinch asafoetida (hing)

1 teaspoon cumin seeds

1 teaspoon freshly grated ginger

ingredients for your dosha (see below) or ½–1 teaspoon curry powder

1–2 tablespoons yellow mung dahl or red lentils, washed 3 times in water

1–2 tablespoons basmati rice, washed 3 times in water

1 cup fresh vegetables, chopped to fit in a thermos flask

2 cups water

Celtic sea salt, to taste

Spice variations for your dosha type
Vata

¼ teaspoon fenugreek seeds

¼ teaspoon fennel seeds

½ teaspoon brown sugar

1 tablespoon yoghurt

Pitta

1 tablespoon sesame seeds

1 tablespoon coconut (shredded or dessicated)

1 teaspoon fennel seeds

1 teaspoon turmeric

1 teaspoon raw sugar

½ teaspoon cinnamon

1 tablespoon currants

Kapha

1 teaspoon mustard (brown or yellow) seeds
½ teaspoon dried chilli or chilli paste or hot curry powder

- ⊚ Heat the oil in a small saucepan and when hot, add a pinch of asafoetida, which will form into tiny bubbles.
- ⊚ Gently fry the spices for 30 seconds, adding seeds first, fresh spices and ginger next and powders last, before adding the rest of the ingredients. Cover well with water and boil for 2–5 minutes. Without wasting time, spoon the boiling hot mixture into a 1-litre open-mouthed thermos flask. Screw the lid on quickly and leave closed for about four hours. The meal will be freshly cooked and ready to eat by lunchtime.

Body type variations

Vata: Add fenugreek seeds after cumin seeds and fry briefly. If fried for too long, they become very bitter and can ruin a meal! Good vegetables to pacify Vata dosha include carrots, radish and sweet potato. Add yoghurt to thermos flask just before serving.

Pitta: Lightly roast sesame seeds, coconut and fennel in the oil along with the cumin and ginger as described above, before adding the vegetables, turmeric, sugar, cinnamon and the currants. Good vegetables to pacify Pitta dosha include pumpkin, sweet potato, zucchini, carrots and English spinach.

Kapha: Add mustard seeds to hot oil first, then cover the saucepan till they pop. Then proceed as described above. Good vegetables to pacify Kapha dosha include cauliflower, cabbage, corn, peas and English spinach.

Glossary

abhyanga – oil massage

agni – digestive fire

asana – yoga posture

ascendant – rising sign in a birth chart

bhakti yoga – the yoga of devotion

bodhisattva – a fully awakened being who devotes their life to the welfare of all sentient beings

chakra – energy centre in the pranic body

dahl – lentil soup popular in the subcontinent

dharma – path through life that supports you and your community

dosha – motivating principle, energy

ghee – clarified butter

guru – teacher

jaggary – dried sugar cane juice

jnana yoga – the yoga of wisdom

jyotish – Vedic astrology

Karma yoga – the yoga of selfless action

kizhi – a pouch full of herbs used in oil massages to reduce inflammation in the body

khichari – rice and lentil dish

kosha – sheath

Lakshmi – Goddess of abundance in India

langhana – fasting

laddu – Indian sweet

masala – spice mixture

mantra – subtle sound used as a focus in meditation

marma – vital point where the physical body and pranic body meet

meridian – channel for the flow of qi or subtle energy

nadi – channel for the flow of prana or subtle energy

nawarakidhi – rice pudding massage

neem – medicinal tree with bitter leaves, used in India

padabhyanga – foot massage

prana – life force, subtle energy

pranayama – yogic breathing exercise designed to control the flow of prana

panchakarma – five deep-cleansing practices described in Ayurveda

permaculture – an approach to agriculture that emphasises biodiversity and sustainability

pizichile – oil bath in which 2 litres of warm oil is massaged into the body

qigong – movement and breathing exercise from traditional Chinese medicine

raja yoga – the yoga of the mystic, literally yoga of the kings

rasayana – science of rejuvenation

reflexology – the art of foot massage where reflex points on the feet are stimulated to induce deep relaxation and healing in the whole body

reiki – a form of spiritual healing

sadhana – spiritual practice

sangha – spiritual community

satsang – company of the wise or truthful

shirodhara – a deeply relaxing oil massage where warm oil is poured in a steady stream over your forehead

swasthavrtta – preventive medicine, habits of self-care

tulsi – sacred basil

vaastu – the science of space, Vedic feng shui including Vedic architecture and sculpture

yatra – pilgrimage

yoga nidra – deep relaxation and meditation practice done lying down

Further reading

Ananth, Sashikala, *The Penguin Guide to Vaastu*, Penguin, New Delhi, 1998.

Ananth, Sashikala, *Vaastu: A Path to Harmonious Living*, Roli Books, New Delhi, 2001.

Brown, Dennis and Jonathan Pedder, *Introduction to Psychotherapy*, Routledge, London, 1979.

Dash, Bhagwan and Manfred Junius, *A Handbook of Ayurveda*, Concept Publishing, New Delhi, 1983.

de Fouw, Hart and Robert Svoboda, *Light on Life*, Lotus Press, Wisconsin, 1996.

Feuerstein, Georg, *The Shambala Encyclopedia of Yoga*, Shambala, Boston and London, 1997.

Kabat-Zinn, *Full Catastrophe Living*, Bantam, New York, 1991.

Frawley, David, *Yoga and Ayurveda*, Lotus Press, Winsconsin, 1999.

Frawley, David, *Ayurveda and the Mind*, Lotus Press, Wisconsin, 1997.

Frawley, David and Vasant Lad, *The Yoga of Herbs*, Lotus Press, New Mexico, 1986.

Frawley, David and Subhash Ranade, *Ayurveda: Nature's Medicine*, Lotus Press, Wisconsin, 2001.

Gawler, Ian, *Peace of Mind*, Michelle Anderson Publishing, Melbourne, 1987.

Hanh, Thich Nhat, *Peace is Every Step*, Bantam, New York, 1991.

Hospodar, Miriam K, *Heaven's Banquet: Vegetarian Cooking for Lifelong Health the Ayurveda Way*, Plume, New York, 2001.

Levine, Stephen, *Who Dies?*, Doubleday, New York, 1982.

Lad, Usha and Dr Vasant Lad, *Ayurvedic Cooking for Self-Healing*, The Ayurvedic Press, Albuqerque, 1994.

Lad, Vasant, *Ayurveda: The Science of Self-Healing*, Lotus Press, Winsconsin, 1984.

Mascaro, Juan (translator), *The Upanishads*, Penguin, London, 1965.

Matthews, Shaun, *Journeys in Healing*, Finch Publishing, Sydney, 2003.

Michie, David, *Hurry Up and Meditate*, Allen and Unwin, 2010, Sydney.

Morningstar, Amadea with Urmila Desai, *The Ayurvedic Cookbook*, Lotus Press, Wisconsin, 1990.

Morningstar, Amadea with Urmila Desai, *Ayurvedic Cooking for Westerners*, Lotus Press, Wisconsin, 1996.

Morrison, Judith, *The Book of Ayurveda*, Simon and Schuster, Sydney, 1995.

Radhakrishnan, S, *The Bagavagita*, Aquarian, London, 1995.

Reid, Linda, *Astrology: Step by Step*, Canopus Publications, Tasmania, 1999.

Saraswati, Swami Satyananda, *Asana, Pranayama, Mudra, Bandha*, Rudra Press, Bihar School of Yoga, Bihar, 1996.

Sharma, PV, *Charaka Samhita*, Chaukhambha Orientalia, Delhi, 1981.

Singer, Peter and Jim Mason, *The Ethics of What We Eat*, Text Publishing, Melbourne, 2006.

Sivan, Pandit Ram, *Hinduism for Beginners*, Simha Publications, Sydney, 1997.

Sri Nisargadatta Maharaj, *I Am That*, Chetana Press, Bombay, 1973.

Sri Ramana Maharshi, *Talks with Sri Ramana Maharshi*, Sri Ramanashramam, Tiruvannamalai, 1955.

Svoboda, Robert, *Prakruti: Your Ayurvedic Constitution*, Geocom, New Mexico, 1989.

Svoboda, Robert, *Ayurveda: Life, Health and Longevity*, Penguin Books, London, 1992.

Vivekananda, Swami, *Raja Yoga*, Advaita Ashrama, Calcutta, 1990.

Vivekananda, Swami, *Karma Yoga*, Advaita Ashrama, Calcutta, 1991.

Vivekananda, Swami, *Jnana Yoga*, Advaita Ashrama, Calcutta, 1989.

Vivekananda, Swami, *Bhakti Yoga*, Advaita Ashrama, Calcutta, 1988.

Resources

Australia and New Zealand

Anahata Therapies (www.anahatatherapies.com.au): Ayurvedic consultations and massage treatments, Sydney

Aspects of Healing (www.aspectsofhealing.com.au) Ayurvedic consultations and treatments, Adelaide

Australasian Association of Ayurveda (AAA) (www.ayur.org.au): Practitioners and treatments, Adelaide

Australasian Institute of Ayurvedic Studies (www.aiasinstitute.com): Courses, practitioners and treatments, Auckland.

Australian Institute of Holistic Medicine (www.aihm.com.au): Advanced Diploma course in Ayurveda, Perth

Ayurveda Elements (www.ayurvedaelements.com): Certificate courses and Ayurvedic consultations, Sydney

Ayurvedic Healing (www.ayurvedichealing.com.au): Ayurvedic consultations and Ayurvedic courses, Sydney

Ayurveda Village (www.ayurvedavillage.com.au): Ayurvedic consultations and treatments, Adelaide Hills

Ayurvedic Wellness Centre (www.ayurvedicwellnesscentre.com.au): Ayurvedic consultations and massage treatments, Sydney

Eumundi Medicine Man (www.eumundimedicineman.com.au): Ayurvedic consultations, massage treatments and herbs, Eumundi, Queensland

EQUALS International (www.equals.edu.au): Advanced Diploma and Certificate IV courses in Ayurveda, Adelaide

Nature Care College (www.naturecare.com.au): Introductory and certificate courses in Ayurveda, Sydney

Planet Ayurveda (www.planetayurveda.co.nz): Ayurveda courses, Australia and New Zealand

Subtle Energies (www.subtleenergies.com.au): Diploma courses in Ayurvedic aromatherapy, consultations and massage treatments, Sydney

Sydney Ayurvedic Centre (www.sydneyayurveda.com): Consultations and treatments, Sydney

The Mudita Institute (www.muditainstitute.com): Ayurvedic consultations, massage treatments and retreats, Byron Bay

Wellpark College (www.wellpark.co.nz): Ayurveda courses in Ayurveda, Auckland, New Zealand

UK, USA and other parts of the world

American Institute of Vedic Studies (www.vedanet.com): Correspondence courses in Ayurveda and Vedic astrology, Santa Fe

Ayurvedic Institute (www.ayurveda.com): Training and online courses in Ayurveda, Albuquerque

Ayurveda Practitioners Association (www.apa.uk.com): Practitioners and continuing professional development courses, UK

California College of Ayurveda (www.ayurvedacollege.com): Training courses in Ayurveda, California

European Institute of Vedic Studies (www.ayurvedicnutrition.com): Ayurvedic training, Europe

Ayurvedic cooking

Joe Harrop (greatgoona@westnet.com.au): Ayurvedic catering and Ayurvedic cookbooks, Sydney

Tim Mitchell (www.yogaofthekitchen.com): Courses in Ayurvedic cooking and Vedic meditation in Australia and Europe

Ayurvedic herbs, teas and oils

Arya Vaidya Pharmacy (www.avpayurveda.com): Based in Coimbatore, south India has excellent Ayurvedic herbal supplies and medicated herbal oils

Banyan Botanicals (www.banyanbotanicals.com): A wide variety of Ayurvedic herbs and products that are sustainably sourced and fairly traded

Pukka herbal teas (www.pukkaherbs.com): Well-crafted organic herbal teas using Ayurvedic principles

A note about the oral traditions of learning

For readers interested in applying the principles of wisdom traditions to their everyday lives, it is important to acknowledge that Ayurveda, Yoga and Vedic astrology are oral traditions. In common with indigenous traditions of learning the world over, they are systems of knowledge that have been passed down from teacher to student over thousands of years. The relationship between the student and teacher is at the very heart of these traditions. It is generally held that progress on the path of integration requires both practise and the guidance of a well-qualified and respected teacher.

In India, the approach to learning is quite different to the approach that has been dominant in the West. In India there is more emphasis on subjective experience. Keen observation using your five senses, tuning into your intuition and making inferences based on your lived experience, are encouraged.

Authoritative statements made by wise and experienced teachers are listened to carefully and contemplated, even if they may, at first, appear to lack adequate explanation. Rather than dismiss them out of hand, the student is advised to accept the point of view initially and then see whether it marries with their experience over time, or not. Some Western students find this approach to learning very challenging.

The oral tradition of learning is alive and well in India today. It is not uncommon to find families who have been practising Ayurveda for over 400 years continuously and sometimes longer. Importantly these traditions recognise that how they are practised needs to be modified according to the time and context. For example, an approach that may have worked well in ancient India may not be appropriate in a Western setting in the 21st century.

Ayurveda also draws from a number of ancient texts, the oldest being the *Rg Veda*, one of humanity's earliest written documents. While there is considerable disagreement regarding when many of these texts were written, it would seem that the *Rg Veda* first appeared at least around 1500 BCE. *Charaka Samhita*, the most well-known textbook of Ayurvedic medicine, is thought to date back to around 500 BCE.

The oldest of the *Upanishads*, which form the basis of Yogic philosophy, is thought to date back to 800 to 600 BCE, while the *Bhagavad Gita*, which extols the virtues of Yoga in detail, is held to have been written around 400 BCE. When it comes to Jyotish or Vedic astrology, the *Rg Veda* includes references to it, though the first texts of astrology appeared around the second century CE in India.

English translations and commentaries of these ancient texts are now freely available on the internet. As well, there are more and more Western teachers, well versed in these traditions of wellbeing, teaching in schools of yoga and meditation, and in Ayurvedic colleges. If you would like to know more, the Resources Section at the back of this book includes the names of a number of well-reputed Ayurvedic centres and colleges outside of India.

Acknowledgements

This book has been enriched by the contributions of many people.

First and foremost I want to wholeheartedly thank all the individuals who shared their stories so generously for this book and who have helped to bring the essence of these ancient approaches to wellbeing alive. In particular, I would like to acknowledge the contributions of Sue Smiles, Davina Chan, Lisa Spinadel, Janet Stratham, Anna Wilson and Lindy Anderson.

I would also like to acknowledge and thank my lecturers and professors at Gujarat Ayurved University for their warm hospitality during my student days in Jamnagar and for generously sharing their knowledge. Heather Farlow for her steadfast encouragement with the writing of this book. It did help keep things moving along. The late, Dr Peter Broughton, for his warm support of my writing and of this book in particular. Carol Marando, Joan Collins and Kylie Hitchman who read some of the early manuscripts of the book. Their generous feedback and comments were very valuable and helped me expand the scope of the book.

Geoff Marx, my astrology teacher, for reviewing the chapter on astrology. His helpful suggestions were most welcome. Tim Mitchell who generously shared some of his fabulous recipes from our Ayurvedic cooking classes. Roland Fishman provided much wise counsel on the writing process at several important points in the book's development. His comments were always very affirming and his unique observations helped in the shaping of the book. Dr Rama Prasad for reviewing chapters 9 and 10 of the book and for his insightful suggestions. Rama has been an invaluable Ayurvedic mentor for me over the years and his counsel on all things Ayurvedic is most appreciated. Farida Irani whose generosity of spirit helped enormously in the final stages of putting this book together and who has been an inspiring and passionate advocate for Ayurveda over many years.

The team at the Ayurvedic Wellness Centre have always been very positive about the writing of this book. Their treatments helped keep my Vata dosha balanced. I would like to give a special thanks to Binu for his magical abhyanga treatments. My partner, Lisa Spinadel, whose ready ear and support of this book never waivered and who has been with me at every step of the way. My son, Bodhi, for his help as a food taster of my culinary experiments and for calmly taking his father's idiosyncrasies in his stride. Jenny Scepanovic for her fine edit and Meg Dunworth for her excellent graphic design work and illustrations.

Finally I am indebted to Rex Finch, Samantha Miles and Laura Boon at Finch Publishing. They have been a delight to work with right from the very inception of this project. Their insightful, creative and practical suggestions have enhanced the book immeasurably. I always had the feeling that the book would be so much the better for their involvement and so it has been.

Other great books from Finch Publishing

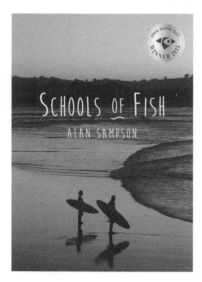

Schools of Fish
Alan Sampson
ISBN:9781925048452

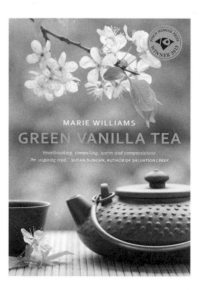

Green Vanilla Tea
Mare Williams
ISBN:9781921462993

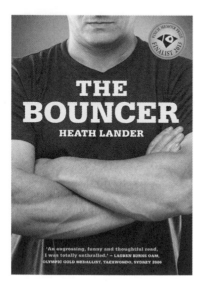

The Bouncer
Heath Lander
ISBN:9780987419651

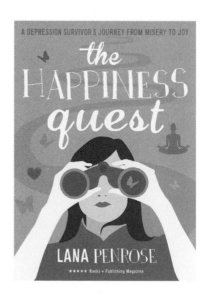

The Happiness Quest
Lorna Penrose
ISBN: 9781925048339